COLLINS GEM

CALORIE COUNTER

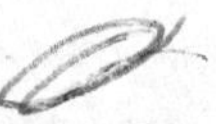

HarperCollins*Publishers*

HarperCollins Publishers
P. O. Box, Glasgow G4 0NB

First published 1984
Fifth edition 1995

Reprint 10 9 8 7 6 5

ISBN 0 00 470735 4

Printed and bound in Great Britain by
Caledonian International Book Manufacturing Ltd, Glasgow, G64

PREFACE TO THE FIFTH EDITION

Since its first publication in 1984, the *Collins Gem Calorie Counter* has firmly established itself as one of the most successful and popular reference guides available for weight watchers.

The text for this edition has been completely revised and updated. Included is data on the amount of Calories contained in a wide range of branded foods, as well as figures for the amount of protein, carbohydrate, fat and dietary fibre in the products covered. Doctors and nutritionists agree that combining these ingredients in the correct proportions is essential to ensure a healthy diet.

The inclusion of this information makes the *Collins Gem Calorie Counter* more than ever the ideal companion for the health-conscious shopper.

INTRODUCTION

For many years, doctors and successful dieters alike have acknowledged that the healthiest and most effective form of weight loss is to combine a Calorie-controlled diet with regular exercise. Now that the body's metabolism is understood more fully, the informed dieter and health-conscious eater wants to know not only the Calorie content of food but also its composition.

The body can be compared to an engine, and the 'fuel' it uses is food. About half the energy provided by food is used to keep the body functioning normally; the other half is taken up by activity such as work and recreation. Generally speaking, active people use more energy and, therefore, need to eat more to meet their energy requirements. If a person consumes more energy than he or she expends, the excess will be stored by the body as fat, and the person will put on weight. Conversely, if a person consumes less energy than he or she expends the extra energy will be taken from the body's fat stores, and the person will lose weight.

The energy provided by food and burnt up by the body is generally measured in Calories, also called kilocalories (kcal). It has been calculated that one pound of body fat is equal to 3500 Calories, so for every pound required to be lost, 3500 Calories must be burnt up or cut out of the diet over several days. On page 13 there is a table which gives the average number of Calories used in an hour taking part in certain activities. However, the rate at which the body uses up Calories varies from person to person, and depends on many factors such as a person's age, sex and general state of fitness, as well as the composition of their diet.

The food that we eat is made up of three major kinds of nutrients: *proteins, carbohydrates* and *fats.* It also provides the body with vitamins and minerals; these are called micronutrients because they are required in much smaller quantities. Nutrients all have important functions within the body.

Proteins are the building bricks of the human body. The cells of our bones, muscles, skin, nails, hair and every other tissue are made up of proteins. Many vital fluids, such as blood, enzymes and hormones, also contain proteins. There is an enormous variety of different kinds of protein, each made up of a special combination of components called amino acids.

The protein in our food is broken down into its component amino acids by the digestive system, and new proteins are synthesized by the body. The best sources of protein in the diet are meat, fish, eggs, milk and other dairy products, corn, lentils and other pulses. The protein obtained from animal sources contains more amino acids than protein from plants. Vegans, therefore, have to eat a wide variety of foods in order to ensure that their diet includes the full complement of amino acids.

Nutritionists recommend that protein represents 10% of the body's daily energy intake. This means that if a person consumes about 2400 Calories a day, 240 of those Calories should be provided by the protein in their food. One gram of protein provides about 4 Calories, so that person needs to consume about 60 grams of protein a day. Many people eat more protein than this, and there is little evidence to suggest that eating too much protein is a health risk. However, a diet low in protein is harmful, particularly to the young who are still growing.

Carbohydrates are made up of different kinds of simple sugars, such as glucose. The scientific name for the sugar that we add to our food is sucrose; one molecule or unit of sucrose is made up of two units of glucose. Carbohydrates can be divided into two different categories. The first category, which we will simply call *carbohydrates*, are known as *available carbohydrates* because the body can obtain energy from them. The second category, usually called *dietary fibres*, are known as *unavailable carbohydrates* because they are indigestible.

Available carbohydrates are important sources of energy for the body. They are broken down by the digestive system into the individual simple sugars; then they can be metabolized immediately to release energy, or they can be converted into fat and put into the body's energy stores. Starch is a form of carbohydrate, and starchy foods – such as wheat, rice, pulses and potatoes – are a good source of carbohydrates. Carbohydrates are also found in fruit and vegetables. Honey, sugar, sweets and sweetened soft drinks contain very high levels of carbohydrates, but they provide the body with virtually no other nutrients. For this reason, energy from these sources is sometimes referred to as 'empty calories'.

Although the body can obtain energy from a diet that contains no carbohydrates, they are still an important part of the diet, not least because foods rich in carbohydrates are usually good sources of micronutrients. For example, grains provide B vitamins, and fruit is an important source of vitamin C. Nutritionists recommend that 50% of the body's energy requirements are derived from carbohydrates. If a person consumes 2400 Calories a day, 1200 of those Calories should be provided by carbohydrates in their food. One gram of carbohydrate provides about 4 Calories, so that person should eat about 300 grams of carbohydrates a day.

Unavailable carbohydrates, or **dietary fibre**, cannot be broken down by the digestive system. Dietary fibre adds bulk to food and contributes to the 'full' feeling after a meal. Although it does not contain any nutrients it is an essential part of the diet and it has a number of beneficial effects, especially assisting the regular and comfortable evacuation of the bowels. Certain kinds of dietary fibre, such as oat bran, are believed to lower levels of cholesterol in the blood. Foods that contain high levels of dietary fibre are, anyway, usually good sources of other nutrients and micronutrients. They include wheat bran and bran cereals, dried fruits, nuts, pulses, and leafy green vegetables.

The average UK diet provides only about 12 grams of dietary fibre a day. Nutritionists recommend that this figure should be nearer 30 grams. If the intake of dietary fibre is increased too rapidly it may cause flatulence and diarrhoea. A very high consumption of fibre may impede the absorption of certain vital minerals.

Fats in food are the perennial enemy of the dieter. Fat has a very high energy value: 1 gram of fat provides 9 Calories; this is more than twice the calorific value of 1 gram of protein or of carbohydrate. The fat obtained from food is only broken down and used as energy when other sources of energy – carbohydrate and protein – have been exhausted. If all the fat in the diet is not converted into energy, it is simply laid down in the body's fat stores. A high intake of fats will, therefore, cause weight gain.

Vegetable oils, dripping, lard, butter, margarine, cream and nuts are all high in fat. Some meats also have a high fat content, but this can usually be reduced by trimming away the visible areas of fat before or after cooking. Fats obtained from animal sources, such as butter and cream, have been associated with an increased risk of coronary heart disease and of cancer if they are consumed in large quantities. Oils obtained from plants do not have this property, and certain vegetable and fish oils are thought to actively reduce the risk of heart disease.

Fat represents about 40% of the total energy intake of the average UK diet. This figure is much higher than it needs to be for the body's requirements. The body needs fat as an energy store and for the formation of cell membranes and the protective sheath that surrounds nerves, as well as the synthesis of certain hormones and enzymes. Most fats can be synthesized from excess carbohydrate and protein, but there are special fats called essential fatty acids which must be obtained from the diet. In order to ensure that these substances are included in the diet, fat should represent at least 2% of the body's energy intake.

However, a diet this low in fat would be unpalatable and difficult to prepare; nutritionists recommend that fat provides about 20% of the daily intake. This means that if a person consumes 2400 Calories a day, 480 of those Calories should be provided by fat in their food. Since 1 gram of fat provides 9 Calories, that person should eat about 53 grams of fat a day.

Among the tables on the following pages are those for desirable weights according to sex, height and frame. These will help to give the dieter a realistic target. Anyone considering trying to lose a lot of weight should consult their doctor, and those just keen not to overdo it should remember that the best way to lose weight – or to maintain a healthy weight – is to eat a balanced diet, to eat in moderation and to take regular exercise.

The foods in this book are listed in **bold type** in strict alphabetical order in the left-hand column of each page, therefore **Crunchy Nut Cornflakes** will come after **Crunchie** which itself follows **Crunch Cakes**. The name of the manufacturer (of branded foods) is given in the second column. The energy value in Calories, the protein, carbohydrate, fat and dietary fibre contents per 100 gram or 100 millilitre are given in the third, fourth, fifth, sixth and seventh columns, respectively. The cross reference ***see individual brands/flavours/types***, e.g. under **Buns**, indicates that data for a particular foodstuff will be listed elsewhere, in this example under **Chelsea Buns, Currant Buns, Hot Cross Buns**, etc. Values for unbranded foods (listed in ***bold italic type***) have been obtained from *The Composition of Foods* (5th edition, 1991) and *Vegetables, Herbs and Spices* (supplement, 1991) by permission of The Royal Society of Chemistry and the Controller of Her Majesty's Stationery Office.

The publishers are grateful to all the manufacturers who gave information on their products. The list of foods included is as up to date as it was possible to make it, but it should be remembered that new food products are frequently put on the market and existing ones withdrawn, so it has not been possible to include everything. If you cannot find a particular food here, you can still, however, obtain guideline figures by finding an equivalent product from a different manufacturer.

Weights and measures

Imperial to Metric

1 ounce (oz) = 28.35 grams (g)
1 pound (lb) = 453.60 grams (g)
1 fluid ounce (fl. oz) = 29.57 millilitres (ml)
1 pint = 0.568 litre

Metric to Imperial

100 grams (g) = 3.53 ounces (oz)
1 kilogram (kg) = 2.2 pounds (lb)
100 millilitres (ml) = 3.38 fluid ounces (fl. oz)
1 litre = 1.76 pints

Average hourly Calorie requirement by activity

	Women	Men
Bowling	207	270
Cycling: moderate	192	256
hard	507	660
Dancing: ballroom	264	352
Domestic work	153	200
Driving	108	144
Eating	84	112
Gardening: active	276	368
Golf	144	192
Ironing	120	160
Office work: active	120	160
Rowing	600	800
Running: moderate	444	592
hard	692	900
Sewing and knitting	84	112
Sitting at rest	84	112
Skiing	461	600
Squash	461	600
Swimming: moderate	230	300
hard	480	640
Table tennis	300	400
Tennis	336	448
Typing	108	144
Walking: moderate	168	224

Desirable weight of adults: small frame

Men									Women								
Height (without shoes)			Weight range						Height (without shoes)			Weight range					
ft	in	m	st	lb	st	lb	kgs	kgs	ft	in	m	st	lb	st	lb	kgs	kgs
5	1	1.55	8	0	8	8	50.8	54.4	4	8	1.42	6	8	7	10	41.7	44.5
5	2	1.58	8	3	8	12	52.2	56.3	4	9	1.45	6	10	7	3	42.6	45.8
5	3	1.60	8	6	9	0	53.5	57.2	4	10	1.47	6	12	7	6	43.6	47.2
5	4	1.63	8	9	9	3	54.9	58.5	4	11	1.50	7	1	7	9	44.9	48.5
5	5	1.65	8	12	9	7	56.3	60.3	5	0	1.52	7	4	7	12	46.3	49.9
5	6	1.68	9	2	9	11	58.1	62.1	5	1	1.55	7	7	8	1	47.6	51.3
5	7	1.70	9	6	10	1	59.9	64.0	5	2	1.58	7	10	8	4	49.0	52.6
5	8	1.73	9	10	10	5	61.7	65.8	5	3	1.60	7	13	8	7	50.4	54.0
5	9	1.75	10	0	10	10	63.5	68.0	5	4	1.63	8	2	8	11	51.7	55.8
5	10	1.78	10	4	11	0	65.3	69.9	5	5	1.65	8	6	9	1	53.5	57.6
5	11	1.80	10	8	11	4	67.1	71.7	5	6	1.68	8	10	9	5	55.3	59.4
6	0	1.83	10	12	11	8	69.0	73.5	5	7	1.70	9	0	9	9	57.2	61.2
6	1	1.85	11	2	11	13	70.8	75.8	5	8	1.73	9	4	10	0	59.0	63.5
6	2	1.88	11	6	12	3	72.6	77.6	5	9	1.75	9	8	10	4	60.8	65.3
6	3	1.91	11	10	12	7	74.4	79.4	5	10	1.78	9	12	10	8	62.6	67.1

Desirable weight of adults: medium frame

Men									Women								
Height (without shoes)			Weight range						Height (without shoes)			Weight range					
ft	in	m	st	lb	st	lb	kgs	kgs	ft	in	m	st	lb	st	lb	kgs	kgs
5	1	1.55	8	6	9	3	53.5	58.5	4	8	1.42	6	12	7	9	43.6	48.5
5	2	1.58	8	9	9	7	54.9	60.3	4	9	1.45	7	0	7	12	44.5	49.9
5	3	1.60	8	12	9	10	56.3	61.7	4	10	1.47	7	3	8	1	45.8	51.3
5	4	1.63	9	1	9	13	57.6	63.1	4	11	1.50	7	6	8	4	47.2	52.6
5	5	1.65	9	4	10	3	59.0	64.9	5	0	1.52	7	9	8	7	48.5	54.0
5	6	1.68	9	8	10	7	60.8	66.8	5	1	1.55	7	12	8	10	49.9	55.3
5	7	1.70	9	12	10	12	62.6	69.0	5	2	1.58	8	1	9	0	51.3	57.2
5	8	1.73	10	2	11	2	64.4	70.8	5	3	1.60	8	4	9	4	52.6	59.0
5	9	1.75	10	6	11	6	66.2	72.6	5	4	1.63	8	8	9	9	54.4	61.2
5	10	1.78	10	10	11	11	68.0	74.8	5	5	1.65	8	12	9	13	56.3	63.1
5	11	1.80	11	0	12	2	69.9	77.1	5	6	1.68	9	2	10	3	58.1	64.9
6	0	1.83	11	4	12	7	71.7	79.4	5	7	1.70	9	6	10	7	59.9	66.7
6	1	1.85	11	8	12	12	73.5	81.7	5	8	1.73	9	10	10	11	61.7	68.5
6	2	1.88	11	13	13	3	75.8	83.9	5	9	1.75	10	0	11	1	63.5	70.3
6	3	1.91	12	4	13	8	78.0	86.2	5	10	1.78	10	4	11	5	65.3	72.1

Desirable weight of adults: large frame

Men									Women								
Height (without shoes)			Weight range						Height (without shoes)			Weight range					
ft	in	m	st	lb	st	lb	kgs	kgs	ft	in	m	st	lb	st	lb	kgs	kgs
5	1	1.55	9	0	10	1	57.2	64.0	4	8	1.42	7	6	8	7	47.2	54.0
5	2	1.58	9	3	10	4	58.5	65.3	4	9	1.45	7	8	8	10	48.1	55.3
5	3	1.60	9	6	10	8	59.9	67.1	4	10	1.47	7	11	8	13	49.4	56.7
5	4	1.63	9	9	10	12	61.2	69.0	4	11	1.50	8	0	9	2	50.8	58.1
5	5	1.65	9	12	11	2	62.6	70.8	5	0	1.52	8	3	9	5	52.2	59.4
5	6	1.68	10	2	11	7	64.4	73.0	5	1	1.55	8	6	9	8	53.5	60.8
5	7	1.70	10	7	11	12	66.7	75.3	5	2	1.58	8	9	9	12	54.9	62.6
5	8	1.73	10	11	12	2	68.5	77.1	5	3	1.60	8	13	10	2	56.7	64.4
5	9	1.75	11	1	12	6	70.3	78.9	5	4	1.63	9	3	10	6	58.5	66.2
5	10	1.78	11	5	12	11	72.1	81.2	5	5	1.65	9	7	10	10	60.3	68.0
5	11	1.80	11	10	13	2	74.4	83.5	5	6	1.68	9	11	11	0	62.1	69.9
6	0	1.83	12	0	13	7	76.2	85.7	5	7	1.70	10	1	11	4	64.0	71.7
6	1	1.85	12	5	13	12	78.5	88.0	5	8	1.73	10	5	11	9	65.8	73.9
6	2	1.88	12	10	14	3	80.7	90.3	5	9	1.75	10	9	12	0	67.6	76.2
6	3	1.91	13	0	14	8	82.6	92.5	5	10	1.78	10	13	12	5	69.4	78.5

Daily Calories for maintenance of desirable weight

Calculated for a moderately active life. If you are very active add 50 Calories; if your life is sedentary subtract 75 Calories.

Weight			Age 18–35		Age 35–55		Age 55–75	
st	lb	kgs	Men	Women	Men	Women	Men	Women
7	1	44.9		1700		1500		1300
7	12	49.9	2200	1850	1950	1650	1650	1400
8	9	54.9	2400	2000	2150	1750	1850	1550
9	2	58.1		2100		1900		1600
9	6	59.9	2550	2150	2300	1950	1950	1650
10	3	64.9	2700	2300	2400	2050	2050	1800
11	0	69.9	2900	2400	2600	2150	2200	1850
11	11	74.8	3100	2550	2800	2300	2400	1950
12	8	79.8	3250		2950		2500	
13	5	84.8	3300		3100		2600	

Abbreviations used in the Tables

g	gram
kcal	kilocalorie
ml	millilitre
N	the nutrient is present in significant quantities but there is no accurate information on the amount
n/a	not available
Tr	trace (less than 0.1g present)

A

Product	*Brand*	*Calories kcal*	*Protein (g)*	*Carbo-hydrate (g)*	*Fat (g)*	*Dietary Fibre (g)*
AB Apricot & Mango Yogurt	Holland & Barrett	118	5.2	17.6	3.0	0.2
Abbey Crunch Biscuits	McVitie's	479	6.1	73.1	18.0	2.6
AB Honey & Almonds Yogurt	Holland & Barrett	120	5.4	16.8	3.5	0.2
AB Natural Yogurt	Holland & Barrett	92.3	6.1	9.1	3.5	n/a
AB Peach & Guava Yogurt	Holland & Barrett	115	5.2	16.8	3.0	0.2
Advocaat		272	4.7	28.4	6.3	nil

All amounts given per 100g/100ml unless otherwise stated

Product	*Brand*	*Calories kcal*	*Protein (g)*	*Carbo-hydrate (g)*	*Fat (g)*	*Dietary Fibre (g)*
Aero Chocolate Drinks, all flavours	Nestlé	97.0	4.6	12.4	3.2	0.2
Aero Minibars	Nestlé	527	8.2	54.5	30.7	n/a
Aero Mousses, all flavours	Chambourcy	211	6.1	27.4	8.6	0.1
After Eight Mints	Nestlé	409	1.8	76.0	13.0	n/a
Alabama Chocolate Fudge Cake	McVitie's	373	4.4	61.5	12.5	0.8
Aladdin Spaghetti Shapes in Tomato Sauce	Heinz	67.0	2.3	13.5	0.4	0.8
Albert's Victorian Chutney	Baxters	145	0.9	37.1	0.2	2.2
Alfredo Choice Dry Mix, as sold	Crosse & Blackwell	400	15.6	59.7	11.2	2.7
All-Bran	Kellogg's	270	14.0	46.0	3.5	24.0
All Butter Shorties, each	Mr Kipling	135	1.2	15.4	7.6	n/a
All Juice Lemonade	Cawston Vale	44.0	Tr	11.7	Tr	n/a
All Sauce	HP	100	1.1	27.0	0.5	n/a

Almonds, flaked/ground		612	21.1	6.9	55.8	12.9
Almond Slice	California Cake & Cookie Ltd	371	12.6	50.8	17.1	n/a
each	Mr Kipling	133	2.2	20.0	4.9	n/a
Almond Yorkie	Nestlé	547	10.5	48.8	34.4	n/a
Alpen	Weetabix	364	10.2	65.5	6.8	7.6
no added sugar	Weetabix	363	12.6	62.1	7.2	7.8
Alphabetti Spaghetti in Tomato Sauce	Crosse & Blackwell	60.0	1.7	12.5	0.4	0.4
Alphabites, baked or grilled, 1oz/28g	Birds Eye	60.0	1.0	9.0	2.0	0.7
Amber Sugar Crystals	Tate & Lyle	398	Tr	99.5	nil	nil
Ambrosia Products: ***see Rice, Sago, etc.***						
American Barbecue Beef Beanfeast, per packet	Batchelors	419	22.4	75.1	5.3	n/a
American Brownies	California Cake & Cookie Ltd	392	4.2	42.8	20.0	0.6

Product	*Brand*	*Calories kcal*	*Protein (g)*	*Carbo-hydrate (g)*	*Fat (g)*	*Dietary Fibre (g)*
American Cajun BBQ Sauce	Campbell's	67.0	1.1	16.4	0.3	n/a
American Cheese & Broccoli Cup-A-Soup, per sachet	Batchelors	131	2.7	18.1	4.9	n/a
American Crisp	Mornflake	474	10.9	68.4	17.4	7.7
American Ginger Ale	Schweppes	22.0	n/a	5.3	n/a	n/a
American Potato & Leek Chowder Soup of the World	Knorr	354	8.0	57.8	10.1	n/a
American Shoofly Pie	California Cake & Cookie Ltd	440	5.5	68.0	19.1	6.5
Anchovies canned in oil, drained		280	25.2	nil	19.9	nil
Anchovy Essence	Burgess	150	13.3	nil	10.4	nil
Anchovy Paste	Shippams	137	19.7	3.2	5.0	n/a
Angel Delight, all flavours, per serving, as sold	Bird's	485	2.5	71.5	21.0	nil
Angel Delight, sugar free, all flavours, as sold	Bird's	490	5.4	58.0	26.0	nil

Animal Bar	Nestlé	512	6.5	61.8	26.5	n/a
Animal Biscuits	Cadbury	493	6.6	70.4	20.6	2.1
Apple & Blackberry Hot Cake	McVitie's	306	3.8	41.8	14.3	1.3
Apple & Blackcurrant Drink, diluted	Quosh	25.0	n/a	6.8	n/a	n/a
Apple & Blackcurrant Drink, per pack	Boots Shapers	55.0	n/a	n/a	Tr	n/a
Apple & Blackcurrant Drink, ready to drink	Quosh	17.0	Tr	4.1	Tr	n/a
Apple & Blackcurrant Juice, diluted	Robinsons	48.0	0.1	11.0	Tr	n/a
Apple & Blackcurrant Individual Pies, each	Mr Kipling	472	3.7	78.4	16.0	n/a
Apple & Blackcurrant Pies, each	Mr Kipling	212	2.1	38.0	8.5	n/a
Apple & Blackcurrant Ready to Drink Carton	Robinsons	47.0	Tr	12.0	Tr	n/a

All amounts given per 100g/100ml unless otherwise stated

Product	Brand	Calories kcal	Protein (g)	Carbo-hydrate (g)	Fat (g)	Dietary Fibre (g)
Apple & Blackcurrant Special R						
ready to drink carton	Robinsons	4.9	Tr	0.8	Tr	n/a
diluted	Ribena	10.0	0.1	1.4	Tr	n/a
Apple & Custard Pies, each	Mr Kipling	254	2.4	37.5	10.1	n/a
Apple & Damson Low Fat Yogurt	Holland & Barrett	97.0	5.4	16.9	0.8	0.2
Apple & Mango Drink, per pack	Boots Shapers	670	n/a	n/a	Tr	n/a
Apple & Raisin Carnation Slender Plan Bars	Nestlé	350	10.8	52.1	12.2	8.8
Apple & Raisin Harvest Chewy Bar, each	Quaker	94.0	1.4	15.5	2.6	0.8
Apple & Raspberry Juice Drink, diluted	Robinsons	48.0	0.1	20.0	Tr	n/a
Apple & Sour Cherry Juice	Cawston Vale	44.0	0.1	10.8	Tr	n/a

Apple & Strawberry Drink Ready to Drink Carton	Robinsons	48.0	Tr	12.0	Tr	n/a
Apple & Strawberry Juice	Copella	39.0	n/a	10.1	nil	Tr
Apple & Strawberry Juice Drink, diluted	Robinsons	88.0	Tr	21.0	Tr	Tr
Apple 'C'	Libby	47.0	Tr	11.7	Tr	nil
Apple Chews, each	Trebor Bassett	15.4	Tr	3.2	0.2	nil
Apple Chutney		201	0.9	52.2	0.2	1.2
Apple Crumble	McVitie's	252	3.3	41.8	8.4	0.9
Apple Crush	Jusoda	31.0	n/a	9.5	Tr	Tr
Apple Drink, Sparkling	St Clements	47.0	n/a	11.6	Tr	Tr
Apple Fruit Juice	Del Monte	43.0	0.1	11.1	Tr	n/a
Apple Juice	Britvic 55	46.0	Tr	11.0	Tr	n/a
	Copella	39.0	n/a	10.1	nil	Tr
unsweetened		38.0	0.1	9.9	0.1	Tr
Apple Juice Drink, diluted	Robinsons	88.0	Tr	21.0	Tr	n/a

All amounts given per 100g/100ml unless otherwise stated

Product	*Brand*	*Calories kcal*	*Protein (g)*	*Carbo-hydrate (g)*	*Fat (g)*	*Dietary Fibre (g)*
Apple Low Calorie Drink						
in bottles	Tango	4.0	Tr	0.8	Tr	n/a
in cans	Tango	5.0	Tr	1.0	Tr	n/a
Apple, Nut & Raisin Yogurt, per pack	Boots Shapers	59.0	n/a	n/a	0.4	n/a
Apple Pashka	McVitie's	244	4.4	26.8	13.5	0.6
Apple Pies	Lyons Bakeries	369	3.1	55.5	15.0	1.2
	McVitie's	235	2.8	35.3	9.6	0.9
each	Mr Kipling	257	2.2	41.2	9.2	n/a
individual, each	Mr Kipling	479	3.5	80.2	16.0	n/a
Apple Rice	Ambrosia	96.0	3.3	15.5	2.7	n/a
Apple Rings	Holland & Barrett	263	2.0	68.0	Tr	12.5
Apple Roll	Jacob's	371	4.1	73.3	6.8	2.7
Apples, cooking						
raw, peeled		35.0	0.3	8.9	0.1	2.2
stewed with sugar		74.0	0.3	19.1	0.1	1.8
stewed without sugar		33.0	0.3	8.1	0.1	1.8

Apples, eating, average, raw		47.0	0.4	11.8	0.1	2.0
Apple Sauce	Colman's	167	0.1	40.0	Tr	n/a
	Heinz	61.0	0.3	14.5	0.2	1.5
Apple Sauce Mix	Knorr	379	0.5	86.9	3.3	n/a
Apple Sauce Spice Cake	California Cake & Cookie Ltd	310	2.0	59.6	7.6	1.3
Apple Sultana Bran Muffin	California Cake & Cookie Ltd	319	4.3	89.7	12.0	7.3
Apple with Apple & Cinnamon Sauce Sponge Pudding	Heinz	278	2.5	44.3	10.0	0.9
Apricot & Almond Frusli Bar	Jordans	429	6.3	64.4	16.2	4.0
Apricot & Mango Extrafruit Yogurt	Ski	94.0	4.9	17.5	0.7	1.0
Apricot & Mango Yogurt	St Ivel Shape	42.0	4.5	5.9	0.1	0.1
Apricot & Raisin Flapjacks, each	Mr Kipling	154	1.5	18.9	8.0	n/a

All amounts given per 100g/100ml unless otherwise stated

Product	*Brand*	*Calories kcal*	*Protein (g)*	*Carbo-hydrate (g)*	*Fat (g)*	*Dietary Fibre (g)*
Apricot & Starfruit Yogurt	St Ivel Shape	41.0	4.5	5.6	0.1	0.1
Apricot & Sultana Stuffing Mix	Knorr	340	10.6	57.4	7.6	n/a
Apricot Chutney	Sharwood	141	1.0	33.9	0.1	4.3
Apricot Fromage Frais per pack	St Ivel Shape	43.0	6.2	4.4	0.1	0.2
	Boots Shapers	108	n/a	n/a	3.9	n/a
Apricot Halves in Syrup	Del Monte	73.0	0.4	18.5	0.2	n/a
	Libby	74.0	0.4	18.0	Tr	0.4
Apricot Jam reduced sugar	Baxters	210	Tr	53.0	nil	1.1
	Heinz Weight Watchers	126	0.2	31.3	nil	0.4
	Holland & Barrett	140	0.5	36.0	nil	nil
Apricot Lightly Whipped Yogurt	St Ivel Prize	133	4.3	14.9	6.4	n/a
Apricot Relish	Colman's	199	1.1	46.0	0.7	n/a

Apricot Rice	Ambrosia	99.0	3.3	16.4	2.7	n/a
Apricots, raw		31.0	0.9	7.2	0.1	1.4
canned in syrup		63.0	0.4	16.1	0.1	1.2
canned in juice		34.0	0.5	8.4	0.1	1.2
Apricot Sucrose Free Jam	Dietade	260	0.3	64.4	Tr	nil
Apricot Sundae Yogurt	St Ivel Shape	41.0	4.5	5.6	0.1	0.1
Aquiesse Citrus Cordial, diluted	Ribena	155	0.1	37.0	Tr	n/a
Aquiesse Mediterranean Cordial, diluted	Ribena	158	0.1	38.0	Tr	n/a
Ardennes Pâté, per pack	Boots Shapers	120	n/a	n/a	7.1	n/a
Aromat	Knorr	178	13.2	24.6	3.0	n/a
Artichoke, globe, raw		18.0	2.8	2.7	0.2	N
boiled		8.0	1.2	1.2	0.1	N
Artichoke, Jerusalem, boiled		41.0	1.6	10.6	0.1	N
Asparagus, raw		25.0	2.9	2.0	0.6	1.7
boiled		13.0	1.6	0.7	0.4	0.7
canned, drained		24.0	3.4	1.5	0.5	2.9

Product	*Brand*	*Calories kcal*	*Protein (g)*	*Carbo-hydrate (g)*	*Fat (g)*	*Dietary Fibre (g)*
Asparagus Slim-A-Soup, per sachet	Batchelors	39.0	1.1	7.1	0.9	n/a
Asparagus Soup, per pack	Boots Shapers	40.00	n/a	n/a	1.3	n/a
Assorted Tools, each	Trebor Bassett	35.0	0.3	0.3	1.9	nil
Aubergine, sliced, fried		302	1.2	2.8	31.9	2.9
Austrian Cream of Herb Soup of the World	Knorr	482	8.8	47.0	28.8	n/a
Avocado Pear, average		190	1.9	1.9	19.5	3.4

B

Baby Button Sprouts	Ross	35.0	4.1	6.6	0.5	3.2
Baby Carrots, 1oz/28g	Birds Eye	7.0	0.2	1.5	Tr	0.5
Baby Sweetcorn: ***see Sweetcorn***						
Bacon, collar joint						
lean & fat, boiled		325	20.4	nil	27.0	nil
lean only, boiled		191	26.0	nil	9.7	nil
Bacon, gammon						
joint, lean & fat, boiled		269	24.7	nil	18.9	nil
joint, lean only, boiled		167	29.4	nil	5.5	nil
Bacon, rashers						
lean only, fried (average)		332	32.8	nil	22.3	nil
lean only, grilled (average)		292	30.5	nil	18.9	nil

Product	Brand	Calories kcal	Protein (g)	Carbo-hydrate (g)	Fat (g)	Dietary Fibre (g)
back , lean & fat, fried		465	24.9	nil	40.6	nil
middle, lean & fat, fried		477	24.1	nil	42.3	nil
middle, lean & fat, grilled		416	24.9	nil	35.1	nil
streaky, lean & fat, fried		496	23.1	nil	44.8	nil
streaky, lean & fat, grilled		422	24.5	nil	36.0	nil
Bacon Crunchy Fries	Golden Wonder	145	2.0	17.7	7.4	0.9
Bacon, Lettuce & Tomato Sandwiches, per pack	Boots Shapers	181	n/a	n/a	n/a	n/a
Bacon, Lettuce & Tomato Club Sandwiches, per pack	Boots Shapers	182	n/a	n/a	n/a	n/a
Bacon Mini Ritz	Jacob's	509	6.7	56.7	28.4	2.0
Bacon Supernoodles, per packet, as served	Batchelors	523	9.1	66.9	24.4	4.7
Bacon Wheat Crunchies	Golden Wonder	180	3.7	20.5	9.3	1.0
Bacon Wotsits, per pack	Golden Wonder	110	1.5	12.1	6.2	0.3
Baked Beans and Beefburgers	HP	93.0	6.1	13.2	1.8	3.7

Baked Beans in tomato sauce		84.0	5.2	15.3	0.6	6.9
	Crosse & Blackwell	75.0	5.0	12.7	0.5	6.0
	Heinz	75.0	4.7	13.6	0.2	3.7
	Holland & Barrett	47.0	2.4	9.0	0.2	1.0
no added sugar	Heinz Weight Watchers	56.0	4.7	8.6	0.2	3.7
with reduced sugar		73.0	5.4	12.5	0.6	7.1
Baked Beans with Bacon	Heinz	91.0	6.0	12.9	1.7	3.0
Baked Beans with Burgerbites	Heinz	103	6.7	12.9	2.8	3.4
Baked Beans with Hotdogs	Heinz	110	5.0	11.1	5.0	2.7
Baked Beans with Low Fat Pork Sausages	Crosse & Blackwell	91.0	6.5	10.2	2.7	5.5
Baked Beans with Mini Sausages	Heinz	117	5.7	13.4	4.5	3.2
Baked Beans with Pepperoni	Heinz	93.0	5.5	13.5	1.9	3.6

All amounts given per 100g/100ml unless otherwise stated

Product	*Brand*	*Calories kcal*	*Protein (g)*	*Carbo-hydrate (g)*	*Fat (g)*	*Dietary Fibre (g)*
Baked Beans with Pork Sausages	Heinz	110	5.0	12.8	4.3	2.7
Baked Beans with Veg. Sausage in Tomato Sauce	Crosse & Blackwell	120	5.3	12.9	5.3	3.6
Baked Potatoes, old, with flesh & skin		136	3.9	31.7	0.2	2.7
Bakers Yeast: ***see Yeast***						
Bakewell Slice, each	Mr Kipling	156	1.4	21.7	7.0	n/a
	Peek Frean	249	6.3	37.5	23.7	1.2
Bakewell Tart	McVitie's	396	5.0	48.9	20.4	0.7
	Mr Kipling	435	3.7	63.8	18.3	n/a
Baking Powder		163	5.2	37.8	Tr	nil
Bamboo Shoots, canned		11.0	1.5	0.7	0.2	1.7
	Sharwood	6.0	0.8	0.3	0.2	1.6
Banana & Toffee Flavour Drink, per pack	Boots Shapers	67.0	n/a	n/a	Tr	n/a
Banana Blancmange Powder,						

as sold	Brown & Polson	339	0.6	82.6	0.7	n/a
Banana Cake	California Cake & Cookie Ltd	328	2.9	60.1	10.0	1.28
Banana Chips	Holland & Barrett	531	2.6	60.9	33.4	1.4
	Whitworths	526	1.0	59.9	31.4	1.7
Banana Crusha	Burgess	115	0.1	28.4	Tr	Tr
Banana, Date & Walnut Muffin	California Cake & Cookie Ltd	372	4.0	51.2	17.8	3.7
Banana Dessert Pot	Ambrosia	101	2.8	15.9	3.0	n/a
Banana Flavour Rice	Ambrosia	101	3.3	16.0	2.7	n/a
Banana Napoli	Lyons Maid	95.0	1.7	10.5	5.1	n/a
Banana Nesquik	Nestlé	394	nil	97.3	0.5	nil
made up with whole milk	Nestlé	168	6.8	18.9	7.8	n/a
with semi-skimmed	Nestlé	131	6.8	18.9	3.7	n/a
ready to drink	Nestlé	68.0	3.2	10.0	1.7	nil
Bananas		95.0	1.2	23.2	0.3	3.1

All amounts given per 100g/100ml unless otherwise stated

Product	*Brand*	*Calories kcal*	*Protein (g)*	*Carbo-hydrate (g)*	*Fat (g)*	*Dietary Fibre (g)*
Banana Split Sundae, per pack	Boots Shapers	87.0	n/a	n/a	4.2	n/a
Banana with Toffee Sauce Sponge Pudding	Heinz	307	2.8	51.1	10.1	0.7
Barbecue Beans	Heinz	90.0	5.1	16.2	0.5	4.2
Barbecue Beef & Tomato Slim-A-Soup Special, per sachet	Batchelors	60.0	1.4	10.6	1.5	n/a
Barbecue Beef Supernoodles, per packet, as served	Batchelors	523	9.1	60.4	24.5	4.7
Barbecue Chicken Mini Bagel, each	Boots Shapers	287	n/a	n/a	n/a	n/a
Barbecue Chicken Sandwiches, per pack	Boots Shapers	242	n/a	n/a	n/a	n/a
Barbecue Cook-In-Sauce	Homepride	81.0	0.7	15.6	1.5	n/a
Barbecued Beef Crisps, per pack	Golden Wonder	152	2.1	12.3	10.5	n/a

Barbecue Mutants	Golden Wonder	90.0	1.2	10.9	4.6	0.2
Barbecue Relish	Burgess	136	1.8	29.3	0.7	1.0
Barbecue Rice & Things	Crosse & Blackwell	370	8.5	76.2	3.5	2.7
Barbecue Sauce		75.0	1.8	12.2	1.8	N
Barley Sugar	Cravens	385	Tr	96.3	nil	nil
each	Trebor Bassett	26.4	nil	6.6	nil	nil
Basil & Oregano Ragu Sauce	Batchelors	30.0	1.9	5.4	0.1	n/a
Basmati Rice	Uncle Ben's	343	9.0	75.5	0.6	n/a
	Whitworths	339	7.4	79.8	0.5	0.5
Bath Oliver (large)	Jacob's	445	9.7	68.3	14.8	2.8
Bath Oliver Biscuits	Fortts	412	8.4	65.5	2.7	
Battenburg Cake	Lyons Bakeries	385	6.1	66.0	10.7	1.1
	Mr Kipling	380	4.2	68.7	9.9	n/a
Battenburg Treats, each	Mr Kipling	176	1.1	27.6	6.8	n/a
Batter Mix, Quick	Whitworths	338	9.3	77.2	1.2	3.7

Product	*Brand*	*Calories kcal*	*Protein (g)*	*Carbo-hydrate (g)*	*Fat (g)*	*Dietary Fibre (g)*
Bavarian Mustard	Colman's	114	5.7	2.6	8.1	n/a
Bavarois Chocolate Dessert	Chambourcy	189	3.8	25.2	8.0	0.3
Bavarois Lemon Dessert	Chambourcy	160	2.4	22.7	6.6	Tr
Bavarois Raspberry Dessert	Chambourcy	162	2.6	25.5	5.5	0.5
Bean & Bacon Soup	Baxters	54.0	1.6	7.0	2.4	1.1
Beanfeast (Batchelors): *see individual flavours*						
Beans: *see types*						
Beans & Bites	Holland & Barrett	90.0	6.8	12.0	2.2	4.0
Beansprouts, mung, raw		31.0	2.9	4.0	0.5	5.6
boiled		25.0	2.5	2.8	0.5	1.3
canned		10.0	1.6	0.8	0.1	0.7
stir fried in oil		25.0	1.9	2.5	6.1	0.9
Beef						
brisket lean & fat, boiled		326	27.6	nil	23.9	nil
forerib, roast		349	22.4	nil	28.8	nil

mince, stewed		229	23.1	nil	15.2	nil
rump steak, lean & fat, fried		246	28.6	nil	14.6	nil
rump steak, lean & fat, grilled		218	27.3	nil	12.1	nil
rump steak, lean only, fried		190	30.8	nil	7.4	nil
rump steak, lean only, grilled		168	28.6	nil	6.0	nil
silverside, lean & fat, boiled		242	28.6	nil	14.2	nil
silverside, lean only, boiled		173	32.3	nil	4.9	nil
sirloin, lean & fat, roast		284	23.6	nil	21.1	nil
sirloin, lean only, roast		192	27.6	nil	9.1	nil
stewing steak, lean & fat, stewed		223	30.9	nil	11.0	nil
topside, lean & fat, roast		214	26.6	nil	12.0	nil
topside, lean only, roast		156	29.2	nil	4.4	nil
Beef & Bacon Hotpot Soup	Heinz	48.0	2.0	7.2	1.2	1.0
Beef & Kidney	Tyne Brand	97.0	10.5	2.0	5.2	n/a
Beef & Kidney Pie	Tyne Brand	154	8.7	13.3	8.1	n/a
Beef & Mushroom Pie	Tyne Brand	162	10.1	11.8	8.3	n/a
Beef & Mushroom with Red Wine	Campbell's	52.0	1.3	3.5	3.7	n/a

Product	*Brand*	*Calories kcal*	*Protein (g)*	*Carbo-hydrate (g)*	*Fat (g)*	*Dietary Fibre (g)*
Beef & Pasta Bake	Findus Dinner Supreme	205	11.3	24.8	6.9	0.4
Beef & Potato Pie	Tyne Brand	191	7.1	22.2	8.2	n/a
Beef & Tomato Bolognese Pasta Soup	Heinz	44.0	1.6	7.1	1.0	0.7
Beef & Tomato Cup-A-Soup, per sachet	Batchelors	72.0	1.2	15.0	1.2	n/a
Beef & Tomato Pot Noodle	Golden Wonder	402	11.9	55.6	14.6	n/a
Beef & Tomato Slim-A-Soup Special, per sachet	Batchelors	56.0	1.9	9.8	1.3	n/a
Beef & Vegetable Pie	Tyne Brand	185	6.5	22.5	7.7	n/a
Beef & Vegetable Soup	Heinz Big Soups	37.0	2.8	6.1	0.6	0.7
	Knorr	293	8.5	57.9	3.0	n/a
Beef Bourguignon Casserole Mix, as sold	Colman's	305	5.4	65.0	1.7	n/a
Beef Broth	Heinz Big Soups	38.0	1.8	6.5	0.6	0.6

	Heinz Farmhouse	45.0	1.5	6.5	1.5	0.2
Beefburgers, fried		264	20.4	7.0	17.3	1.4
100%	Ross	293	17.0	nil	25.0	nil
100%, each	Birds Eye Steakhouse	150	9.0	0.1	9.0	nil
economy	Ross	255	13.6	9.9	18.1	0.4
low fat, each	Birds Eye Steakhouse	85.0	9.0	2.0	4.5	0.1
original, each	Birds Eye Steakhouse	120	0.9	1.5	8.5	0.1
quarter-pounders, each	Birds Eye Steakhouse	235	17.0	3.5	17.0	0.2
Beef Cannelloni	Findus Dinner Supreme	140	6.6	12.7	7.0	0.7
Beef Casserole	Tyne Brand	93.0	6.2	6.5	4.7	n/a
Beef Casserole Microchef Meal	Batchelors	85.0	7.1	7.8	3.0	n/a

Product	*Brand*	*Calories kcal*	*Protein (g)*	*Carbo-hydrate (g)*	*Fat (g)*	*Dietary Fibre (g)*
Beef Chow Mein Pot Meal, per pack	Boots Shapers	157	n/a	n/a	5.9	n/a
Beef Consomme	Baxters	12.0	2.4	0.7	Tr	nil
Beef Curry	Campbell's	95.0	5.8	9.6	3.7	n/a
	Tyne Brand	98.0	5.5	9.2	4.3	n/a
	Vesta	107	3.5	18.8	2.5	n/a
with rice	Heinz Lunch Bowl	84.0	4.1	11.7	2.4	0.6
with rice, per pack	Birds Eye Menu Master	410	24.0	64.0	6.5	2.2
Beef Dripping		891	Tr	Tr	99.0	nil
Beefeater Fast Fry Chips	McCain	101	2.4	17.4	2.4	n/a
Beefeater Oven Chips	McCain	155	2.0	27.5	4.1	n/a
Beef Goulash Casserole Mix, as sold	Colman's	303	6.7	59.0	3.9	n/a
Beef Goulash Microchef Snack	Batchelors	58.0	3.9	8.7	1.1	n/a

Beef Goulash Simply Fix Dry Mix, as sold	Crosse & Blackwell	325	10.1	49.5	9.7	4.8
Beef Goulash with Noodles	Heinz Lunch Bowl	80.0	4.4	10.5	2.2	0.8
Beef Goulash with Parsley Rice Big Deal	Heinz Weight Watchers	91.0	5.2	13.1	2.0	0.3
Beef Grillsteaks, grilled, each	Birds Eye Steakhouse	165	13.0	1.0	12.0	nil
Beef Hotpot, per pack	Birds Eye Menu Master	415	23.0	43.0	17.0	2.1
Beef in Barbecue Sauce Toast Topper	Heinz	93.0	4.6	12.0	2.9	1.1
Beef in Beer Casserole Recipe Sauce	Knorr	44.0	0.7	10.5	0.2	n/a
Beef in Black Bean Sauce Readymeal	Uncle Ben's	85.0	6.3	8.1	3.0	n/a
Beef Julienne	Findus Lean Cuisine	100	7.3	13.2	1.9	0.7

All amounts given per 100g/100ml unless otherwise stated

Product	Brand	Calories kcal	Protein (g)	Carbo-hydrate (g)	Fat (g)	Dietary Fibre (g)
Beef Lasagne	Heinz Weight Watchers	95.0	6.1	10.6	3.2	0.6
Beef Madras Curry	Findus Dinner Supreme	120	6.4	17.1	2.7	0.8
	Vesta	105	3.6	19.4	2.0	n/a
per single serving	Vesta	490	17.4	82.6	10.1	n/a
Beef Madras Curry Simply Fix Dry Mix, as sold	Crosse & Blackwell	326	10.8	49.1	8.7	4.4
Beef Oriental with Special Egg Rice	Heinz	86.0	4.5	12.5	2.0	0.5
Beef Pâté	Shippams	204	17.3	1.5	14.3	n/a
Beef, Potato & Red Pepper Premium Soup	Heinz	48.0	2.3	4.5	2.3	0.5
Beef Risotto	Vesta	152	5.5	22.9	4.9	n/a
per single serving	Vesta	338	12.4	59.6	5.6	n/a
Beef Satay Stir Fry Mix,	Crosse &					

as sold	Blackwell	415	13.0	46.3	19.9	2.3
Beef Sausages: ***see Sausages, beef***						
Beef Savoury Rice, per packet, as served	Batchelors	469	9.9	95.0	5.5	5.6
Beef Seasoning Dry Sauce Mix, as sold	Colman's	327	9.3	68.0	1.6	n/a
Beef Soup	Heinz	400	1.7	4.3	1.8	0.2
Beef Stew		120	9.7	4.6	7.2	0.7
	Campbell's	70.0	5.6	8.5	1.8	1.1
	Tyne Brand	83.0	4.8	7.2	3.8	n/a
Beef Stew & Dumplings	Findus Dinner Supreme	120	7.2	9.2	5.8	1.0
per pack	Birds Eye Menu Master	330	23.0	35.0	11.0	2.8
Beef Stock Cubes	Knorr	318	14.0	25.5	17.8	n/a
Beef Stock Powder	Knorr	203	9.7	29.4	5.2	n/a
Beef Stroganoff	Heinz Weight Watchers	93.0	6.9	10.7	2.3	0.6

Product	*Brand*	*Calories kcal*	*Protein (g)*	*Carbo-hydrate (g)*	*Fat (g)*	*Dietary Fibre (g)*
Beef Stroganoff Casserole Mix, as sold	Colman's	390	16.0	47.0	15.0	n/a
Beef Stroganoff Simply Fix Dry Mix, as sold	Crosse & Blackwell	350	13.5	48.8	11.0	2.2
Beef Wotsits, per pack	Golden Wonder	110	1.6	12.0	6.2	0.3
Beer						
bitter, canned		32.0	0.3	2.3	Tr	nil
bitter, draught		32.0	0.3	2.3	Tr	nil
bitter, keg		31.0	0.3	2.3	Tr	nil
mild, draught		25.0	0.2	1.6	Tr	nil
Beetroot, raw		36.0	1.7	7.6	0.1	2.8
boiled		46.0	2.3	9.5	0.1	2.3
pickled		28.0	1.2	5.6	0.2	2.5
pickled, all varieties	Baxters	35.0	1.8	6.8	Tr	2.5
Beetroot in Redcurrant Jelly	Baxters	167	0.7	43.9	Tr	0.9
Bengal Hot Chutney	Sharwood	200	0.5	48.7	0.3	1.1

Best Burgers	Ross	298	12.7	4.2	25.6	0.2
Best English Mints	Cravens	387	Tr	96.1	0.2	nil
Bhuna Classic Curry	Homepride	74.0	1.9	9.8	3.1	n/a
Biarritz	Cadbury	475	4.0	61.6	23.5	n/a
Big Breakfast, each	McDonald's	631	28.8	41.2	39.0	0.9
Bigga Marrowfat Peas	Batchelors	93.0	6.5	20.2	0.6	n/a
Big Mac, each	McDonald's	486	25.8	36.7	26.2	3.7
Big Soups (Heinz): ***see individual flavours***						
Biscuits						
chocolate, full coated		524	5.7	67.4	27.6	2.9
digestive, chocolate		493	6.8	66.5	24.1	3.1
digestive, plain		471	6.3	68.6	20.9	4.6
sandwich		513	5.0	69.2	25.9	1.1
semi-sweet		457	6.7	74.8	16.6	2.1
short-sweet		469	6.2	62.2	23.4	1.5
Bisto Cheese Sauce Granules, as sold	RHM Foods	592	6.4	38.6	45.8	0.6

All amounts given per 100g/100ml unless otherwise stated

Product	Brand	Calories kcal	Protein (g)	Carbo-hydrate (g)	Fat (g)	Dietary Fibre (g)
made up	RHM Foods	99.0	1.1	6.4	7.6	0.1
Bisto Chicken Gravy Granules,						
as sold	RHM Foods	493	4.0	38.7	36.0	n/a
made up	RHM Foods	37.0	0.3	2.9	2.7	Tr
Bisto Fuller Flavour Gravy						
Granules, as sold	RHM Foods	326	7.3	63.5	3.8	1.0
made up	RHM Foods	480	4.0	42.7	33.3	2.7
Bisto Onion Gravy Granules,						
as sold	RHM Foods	248	1.7	59.8	0.2	n/a
made up	RHM Foods	36.0	0.3	3.2	2.5	0.2
Bisto Original, made up	RHM Foods	16.6	Tr	2.0	Tr	n/a
Bisto Parsley Sauce Granules,						
as sold	RHM Foods	584	3.6	43.4	44.0	0.8
made up	RHM Foods	507	4.4	38.8	36.5	0.4
Bisto Rich Gravy Granules,						
made up	RHM Foods	36.0	0.3	2.8	2.6	Tr

Bitter: ***see Beer***

Bitter Lemon	Schweppes	33.9	n/a	8.3	n/a	n/a
Black Bean & Vegetable Stir Fry Sauce	Uncle Ben's	50.0	1.8	9.0	0.7	n/a
Black Bean Stir Fry Mix, as sold	Crosse & Blackwell	335	10.9	56.9	7.2	2.6
Black Bean Stir Fry Sauce	Sharwood	90.0	0.3	19.9	1.3	1.2
Blackberries, raw		25.0	0.9	5.1	0.2	6.6
stewed with sugar		56.0	0.7	13.8	0.2	5.2
stewed without sugar		21.0	0.8	4.4	0.2	5.6
Blackberry & Apple Crumble	Jacob's	484	6.1	63.6	22.8	2.8
Blackberry & Apple Special R, diluted	Ribena	9.0	0.1	1.2	Tr	n/a
Black Cherries in Syrup	Libby	73.0	n/a	n/a	Tr	n/a
Black Cherry Cheesecake Mix	Green's/ Homepride	259	3.0	35.0	12.0	n/a

All amounts given per 100g/100ml unless otherwise stated

Product	*Brand*	*Calories kcal*	*Protein (g)*	*Carbo-hydrate (g)*	*Fat (g)*	*Dietary Fibre (g)*
Black Cherry Crusha	Burgess	128	nil	37.0	nil	nil
Black Cherry Lightly Whipped Yogurt	St Ivel Prize	137	4.3	15.9	6.4	n/a
Black Cherry Long Life Yogurt	St Ivel Prize	71.0	3.4	14.4	0.1	0.4
Blackcherry Ripple Mousse, each	Fiesta	87.0	2.0	11.6	4.0	n/a
Black Cherry Yogurt	Ski	95.0	5.1	17.3	1.1	nil
	St Ivel Shape	42.0	4.5	5.9	0.1	0.1
Blackcurrant & Apple C-Vit	SmithKline Beecham	144	n/a	38.4	n/a	n/a
Blackcurrant & Apple Drink, per pack	Boots Shapers	nil	n/a	n/a	nil	n/a
Blackcurrant & Apple Juice	Copella	50.0	n/a	12.5	nil	Tr
Blackcurrant & Apple Pies	Lyons Bakeries	378	3.2	56.2	15.6	1.2
Blackcurrant & Liquorice	Cravens	404	0.6	91.4	4.1	nil

Blackcurrant Bio Stirred Yogurt	Ski	109	5.8	16.0	2.9	nil
Blackcurrant 'C'	Libby	54.0	Tr	13.5	Tr	nil
Blackcurrant Cheesecake	Eden Vale	261	2.8	38.8	11.6	n/a
	Heinz Weight Watchers	159	4.4	25.6	4.0	0.6
	McVitie's	296	4.5	31.9	17.1	0.7
Blackcurrant Cordial, diluted	Britvic	22.0	Tr	5.3	Tr	n/a
Blackcurrant Creme Sundae Yogurt	St Ivel Shape	41.0	4.6	5.6	0.1	0.4
Blackcurrant C-Vit	SmithKline Beecham	144	n/a	38.5	n/a	n/a
Blackcurrant Devonshire Cheesecake	St Ivel	262	4.9	28.9	14.3	1.3
Blackcurrant Flavoured Cordial	Quosh	22.0	Tr	5.3	Tr	n/a

All amounts given per 100g/100ml unless otherwise stated

Product	*Brand*	*Calories kcal*	*Protein (g)*	*Carbo-hydrate (g)*	*Fat (g)*	*Dietary Fibre (g)*
Blackcurrant Jam	Baxters	210	Tr	53.0	Tr	3.1
reduced sugar	Heinz Weight Watchers	126	0.3	31.2	nil	1.2
	Holland & Barrett	140	0.5	36.0	nil	nil
Blackcurrant Juice Drink	Ribena	59.0	Tr	15.6	n/a	n/a
undiluted	Ribena	285	Tr	76.0	n/a	n/a
Blackcurrant Juice Ready to Drink Carton	Robinsons	48.0	0.1	13.0	Tr	n/a
Blackcurrant Party Cheesecake	McVitie's	295	4.4	33.8	16.1	0.8
Blackcurrants, raw		28.0	0.9	6.6	Tr	7.8
stewed with sugar		58.0	0.7	15.0	Tr	6.1
canned in juice		31.0	0.8	7.6	Tr	4.2
canned in syrup		72.0	0.7	18.4	Tr	3.6
Blackcurrant Sucrose Free Jam	Dietade	269	0.3	67.0	Tr	n/a

Blackeye Beans, boiled		116	8.8	19.9	0.7	3.5
	Batchelors	107	7.8	22.9	0.8	n/a
Black Forest Fromage Frais	St Ivel Shape	55.0	6.3	6.8	0.3	0.2
Black Forest Gateau	McVitie's	291	2.6	36.1	15.3	0.4
	St Ivel	299	4.1	24.8	20.4	0.4
Black Forest Party Gateau	McVitie's	302	2.7	33.8	17.5	0.5
Black Forest Yogurt	St Ivel Shape	46.0	4.6	6.2	0.2	0.1
Black Jack Chews, each	Trebor Bassett	15.4	nil	3.3	0.2	nil
Black Magic Assortment	Nestlé	455	4.5	62.8	20.6	n/a
Black Pudding, fried		305	12.9	15.0	21.9	0.5
Black Treacle	Lyle's	257	1.0	64.0	nil	nil
Bloater Pâté	Shippams	172	18.0	2.2	10.1	n/a
Blue Band Margarine	Van Den Berghs	740	0.1	0.5	82.0	nil
Blueberry Muffin	California Cake & Cookie Ltd	326	5.6	42.6	15.7	1.8

All amounts given per 100g/100ml unless otherwise stated

Product	*Brand*	*Calories kcal*	*Protein (g)*	*Carbo-hydrate (g)*	*Fat (g)*	*Dietary Fibre (g)*
Blueberry Napoli	Lyons Maid	104	1.8	12.7	5.2	n/a
Blueberry Yogurt Mousse, per pack	Boots Shapers	55.0	n/a	n/a	1.3	n/a
Blue Cheese Dip, per pack	Boots Shapers	145	n/a	n/a	12.0	n/a
Blue Riband Milk	Nestlé	519	6.4	60.4	28.0	n/a
Plain	Nestlé	519	4.5	60.4	28.8	n/a
Blue Stilton Cheese: *see Stilton*						
Boasters	McVitie's	547	6.3	54.8	33.1	1.8
Bodyline Natural Cottage Cheese	Eden Vale	85.0	14.0	4.4	1.5	nil
Bodyline Onion & Chive Cottage Cheese	Eden Vale	105	12.7	4.3	4.0	nil
Bodyline Pineapple Cottage Cheese	Eden Vale	97.0	11.6	5.3	3.5	0.2
Boiled Sweets		327	Tr	87.3	Tr	nil

Bologness Beanfeast, per packet, as served	Batchelors	333	26.9	49.0	4.6	n/a
Bolognese Casserole Recipe Sauce	Knorr	62.0	1.7	7.4	3.0	n/a
Bolognese Pasta Choice	Crosse & Blackwell	385	16.9	60.3	8.1	3.2
Bolognese Pot Pasta	Golden Wonder	349	17.7	59.8	4.4	n/a
Bolognese Ragu Sauce	Batchelors	47.0	1.5	9.8	0.1	n/a
Bolognese Sauce, cooked		145	8.0	3.7	11.1	1.1
	Dolmio	91.0	7.2	7.1	3.8	n/a
Bolognese Sauce, cooked						
with Mushrooms	Buitoni	60.0	3.8	9.5	0.9	0.6
with Peppers	Buitoni	65.0	3.8	9.7	1.0	0.6
with Peppers (no meat)	Buitoni	91.0	1.8	18.7	0.8	0.8
Bolognese Shells Italiana	Heinz Weight Watchers	73.0	5.1	10.0	1.4	0.8

All amounts given per 100g/100ml unless otherwise stated

Product	Brand	Calories kcal	Protein (g)	Carbo-hydrate (g)	Fat (g)	Dietary Fibre (g)
Bombay Mix		503	18.8	35.1	32.9	6.2
	Holland & Barrett	505	33.0	35.0	27.0	8.0
	Sharwood	502	19.1	35.5	32.5	8.4
Bombay Potato Flat Bread, each	Boots Shapers	249	n/a	n/a	n/a	n/a
Bombay Spiced Poppadums	Sharwood	281	23.3	42.9	1.8	12.4
Bon Bons, all flavours, each	Trebor Bassett	28.0	nil	5.8	0.4	nil
Boost	Cadbury	495	6.3	58.7	26.2	n/a
Boots Shapers Products: *see under individual products*						
Borlotti Beans	Napolina	70.0	4.9	12.8	0.3	5.5
Bounty, dark	Mars	481	3.2	57.4	26.5	n/a
milk	Mars	485	4.6	56.4	26.8	n/a
Bourbon Biscuits	Jacob's	464	4.8	66.5	21.7	1.5
Bournville	Cadbury	495	4.6	59.6	26.6	n/a

Bournville Cakes	Mr Kipling	138	1.2	17.6	6.9	n/a
Bournville Cakes with Tia Maria	Mr Kipling	103	0.9	12.4	5.0	n/a
Bournville Chocolate Roll	Mr Kipling	422	4.0	57.1	19.0	n/a
Bournville Selection	Cadbury	475	4.0	61.6	23.5	n/a
Bournvita Powder		341	7.7	79.0	1.5	N
made up with whole milk		76.0	3.4	7.6	3.8	Tr
made up with semi-skimmed milk		58.0	3.5	7.6	1.6	Tr
Boursin au Concombreau	Van Den Berghs	233	7.0	4.0	21.0	Tr
au Poivre	Van Den Berghs	414	7.0	2.0	42.0	Tr
au Roquefort	Van Den Berghs	243	8.5	4.0	21.5	n/a
aux Olives	Van Den Berghs	234	8.0	3.5	21.0	n/a
with Garlic	Van Den Berghs	413	7.3	2.7	41.5	n/a
Bovril		169	38.0	2.9	0.7	nil
Bovril Beef Instant Drink	CPC Foods	286	68.2	3.3	Tr	n/a
Bovril Beef Stock Cubes	CPC Foods	181	29.2	6.8	4.2	n/a
Bovril Chicken Extract	CPC Foods	138	14.2	17.3	1.3	n/a

All amounts given per 100g/100ml unless otherwise stated

Product	Brand	Calories kcal	Protein (g)	Carbo-hydrate (g)	Fat (g)	Dietary Fibre (g)
Bovril Chicken Instant Drink	CPC Foods	272	40.5	20.8	3.0	n/a
Bovril Chicken Stock Cubes	CPC Foods	195	27.1	12.3	4.1	n/a
Boysenberries in Syrup	Libby	68.0	n/a	n/a	Tr	n/a
Braised Beef	Tyne Brand	102	10.9	3.2	5.1	n/a
Bramley Apple Dessert	Mr Kipling	342	3.4	55.8	11.7	n/a
Bramley Apple Hot Cake	McVitie's	314	3.9	43.1	14.6	1.3
Bramley Apple Shortcakes, each	Mr Kipling	165	1.4	22.9	7.4	n/a
Bran, wheat		206	14.1	26.8	5.5	39.6
Bran & Apple Crunchy Cereal	Holland & Barrett	367	12.0	60.0	13.0	15.0
Bran Buds	Kellogg's	280	13.0	51.0	3.0	22.0
Brandy: ***see Spirits***						
Bran Fare	Weetabix	252	17.0	34.4	5.2	34.3
Bran Flakes	Kellogg's	320	11.0	64.0	2.0	13.0

Bran Oatcakes, each	Vessen	57.0	1.5	7.8	2.1	0.9
Branston Fruity Sauce	Crosse & Blackwell	117	0.9	25.6	0.2	1.1
Branston Sandwich Pickle	Crosse & Blackwell	122	0.8	28.0	0.1	1.7
Branston Spicy Sauce	Crosse & Blackwell	115	1.0	23.9	0.7	1.3
Branston Sweet Hot Pickle	Crosse & Blackwell	150	0.7	34.5	0.2	1.7
Brawn		153	12.4	nil	11.5	nil
Brazil Nuts		682	14.1	3.1	68.2	8.1
	Holland & Barrett	619	12.0	4.1	61.5	9.0
Brazil Nut Toffees, each	Trebor Bassett	39.3	0.3	5.2	1.8	nil
Bread (see also types)						
brown		218	8.5	44.3	2.0	5.9
	Heinz Weight Watchers	212	12.1	36.8	1.9	0.5

All amounts given per 100g/100ml unless otherwise stated

Product	Brand	Calories kcal	Protein (g)	Carbo-hydrate (g)	Fat (g)	Dietary Fibre (g)
	Sunblest	220	8.0	44.1	1.3	4.3
brown, toasted		272	10.4	56.5	2.1	7.1
currant		289	7.5	50.7	7.6	3.8
currant, toasted		323	8.4	56.8	8.5	4.2
French stick		270	9.6	55.4	2.7	5.1
granary		235	9.3	46.3	2.7	6.5
malt		268	8.3	56.8	2.4	6.5
pitta, white		265	9.2	57.9	1.2	3.9
rye		219	8.3	45.8	1.7	5.8
wheatgerm		212	9.5	41.5	2.0	5.1
wheatgerm, toasted		271	12.1	53.2	2.6	6.5
white		235	8.4	49.3	1.9	3.8
white, fried in oil/lard		503	7.9	48.5	32.2	3.8
white, toasted		265	9.3	57.1	1.6	4.5
wholemeal		215	9.2	41.6	2.5	7.4
wholemeal, toasted		252	10.8	48.7	2.9	8.7
Breaded Cod Fillets	Ross	180	11.1	17.9	7.4	0.8
Breaded Haddock Fillets	Ross	183	11.6	19.6	6.8	0.8

Breadfruit, canned, drained		66.0	0.6	16.4	0.2	2.5
Bread Pudding		297	5.9	49.7	9.6	3.0
Bread Rolls, brown, crusty		255	10.3	50.4	2.8	7.1
soft		268	10.0	51.8	3.8	6.4
Bread Rolls, white						
crusty		280	10.9	57.6	2.3	4.3
soft		268	9.2	51.6	4.2	3.9
Bread Rolls, wholemeal		241	9.0	48.3	2.9	8.8
Bread Sauce						
made with whole milk		150	4.1	10.9	10.3	0.6
made semi-skimmed milk		128	4.2	11.1	7.8	0.6
Bread Sauce Mix	Colman's	325	12.0	66.0	1.3	n/a
Breakfast Juice	Del Monte	38.0	0.5	9.4	Tr	n/a
Brie Cheese		319	19.3	Tr	26.9	nil
Broad Beans, boiled		48.0	5.1	5.6	0.8	5.4
frozen, boiled		81.0	7.9	11.7	0.6	6.5
canned		77.0	5.9	13.0	0.5	5.2

Product	*Brand*	*Calories kcal*	*Protein (g)*	*Carbo-hydrate (g)*	*Fat (g)*	*Dietary Fibre (g)*
Broccoli, boiled		24.0	3.1	1.1	0.8	2.3
Broccoli & Cauliflower Packet Soup, as served	Batchelors	439	9.0	58.9	20.4	4.1
Broccoli & Cauliflower Slim-A-Soup Special, per sachet	Batchelors	59.0	1.3	8.4	2.4	n/a
Broccoli & Gruyere Soup	Baxters	56.0	2.0	4.7	3.3	0.9
Broccoli Mix	Ross	41.0	2.3	9.0	0.5	2.3
Brown Ale, bottled		28.0	0.3	3.0	Tr	nil
Brown Bread: ***see Bread***						
Brown Lentils: ***see Lentils***						
Brown Rice: ***see Rice***						
Brown Ryvita, per slice	Ryvita	25.0	0.7	5.6	0.2	1.3
Brown Sauce, bottled		99.0	1.1	25.2	nil	0.7
	Burgess	97.0	1.1	20.4	0.2	1.0
	Daddies	87.0	1.0	20.0	0.3	n/a

Brown Wheat Cracker	Jacob's	450	9.6	64.4	17.1	3.0
Brussels Sprouts, boiled		35.0	2.9	3.5	1.3	2.6
Bubble & Squeak	Ross	111	1.7	13.8	6.0	1.3
Bulgur	Holland & Barrett	306	10.3	68.0	1.2	6.3
Buns: ***see individual flavours***						
Burger Sauce	Burgess	594	2.1	10.7	59.8	nil
Butter		737	0.5	Tr	81.7	nil
	Kerrygold	720	0.4	Tr	80.0	n/a
Butter Beans, dried, boiled		103	7.1	18.4	0.6	5.2
canned		77.0	5.9	13.0	0.5	4.6
	Batchelors	97.0	8.1	19.1	0.4	3.9
	Holland & Barrett	77.0	5.9	13.0	0.5	4.6
Buttermilk	Raines	40.0	4.3	5.5	0.1	n/a
Buttermint Bonbons	Cravens	425	0.5	86.1	8.7	nil

Product	*Brand*	*Calories kcal*	*Protein (g)*	*Carbo-hydrate (g)*	*Fat (g)*	*Dietary Fibre (g)*
Butter Mintoes	Cravens	425	0.1	86.6	8.7	nil
Butterscotch	Cravens	411	0.1	89.9	5.7	nil
Butterscotch Flavour Pouring Syrup	Lyle's	284	Tr	76.0	nil	Tr
Buttons Cakes	Mr Kipling	112	1.7	13.4	5.3	n/a

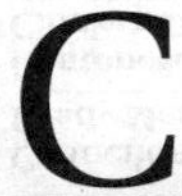

Food	Brand					
***Cabbage**, average, raw*		26.0	1.7	4.1	0.4	2.4
boiled		16.0	1.0	2.2	0.4	1.8
Caerphilly Cheese		375	23.2	0.1	31.3	nil
Cajun Chicken Bap, each	Boots Shapers	194	n/a	n/a	n/a	n/a
Cajun Chicken Big Deal	Heinz Weight Watchers	93.0	4.4	12.8	2.6	0.6
Cajun Chicken Crisps, per pack	Golden Wonder	202	2.9	16.3	13.9	1.8
Cajun Mustard	Colman's	164	6.1	20.0	5.7	n/a
Cajun Sauce	Burgess	175	1.0	33.2	3.5	1.6
Cajun Spicy Vegetable Slim-A-Soup Special, per sachet	Batchelors	55.0	1.6	10.0	1.2	n/a

All amounts given per 100g/100ml unless otherwise stated

Product	*Brand*	*Calories kcal*	*Protein (g)*	*Carbo-hydrate (g)*	*Fat (g)*	*Dietary Fibre (g)*
Cakes with Fruit & Nuts	Mr Kipling	118	1.6	15.6	5.4	n/a
Calabrese: *see Broccoli*						
Calcium Enriched Soya Milk	Holland & Barrett	46.0	3.6	3.3	2.1	Tr
Camembert		297	20.9	Tr	23.7	nil
Cannelini Beans	Batchelors	101	7.6	21.9	0.8	n/a
	Napolina	70.0	4.9	12.9	0.2	5.2
Cannelloni, per pack, low calorie	Heinz Weight Watchers	79.0	3.1	11.8	2.2	1.0
Cannelloni Bistro Break	HP	106	5.2	11.3	4.0	2.9
Cannelloni Bolognese	Dolmio	149	6.1	11.8	8.3	n/a
Cannelloni Cheese & Spinach Ready Meal	Dolmio	125	4.3	8.7	8.1	n/a
Cantonese Sweet & Sour Chicken Dish	Knorr	87.0	0.8	21.8	0.2	0.5

Cappuccino						
instant	Nescafé	386	10.6	62.8	10.3	nil
unsweetened	Nescafé	394	14.2	52.0	14.3	nil
Cappuccino Bar, each	Boots Shapers	98.0	n/a	n/a	4.1	n/a
Capriccio, each	Nestlé	166	2.0	12.5	11.7	n/a
Captain's Cod Pie, per pack	Birds Eye Menu Master	355	25.0	30.0	15.0	1.8
Caramac	Nestlé	545	6.8	56.3	32.5	n/a
Caramac Breakaway	Nestlé	517	7.1	58.8	28.2	n/a
Caramac Ice Cream, each	Nestlé	144	2.0	15.2	8.2	n/a
Caramel	Cadbury	495	5.3	63.6	24.2	n/a
Caramel & Walnut Cake	McVitie's	317	3.5	36.9	17.5	0.7
Caramel Bar, each	Boots Shapers	97.0	n/a	n/a	3.7	n/a
Caramel Cakes, each	Cadbury	90.1	1.1	120	3.9	n/a
Caramel Flavour Rice	Ambrosia	100	3.3	16.0	2.7	n/a

Product	*Brand*	*Calories kcal*	*Protein (g)*	*Carbo-hydrate (g)*	*Fat (g)*	*Dietary Fibre (g)*
Caramel Granymels	Itona	385	0.8	69.0	13.2	n/a
Caramel Hot Chocolate, per pack	Boots Shapers	40.0	n/a	n/a	0.9	n/a
Caramel Log	Tunnock's	472	4.2	64.3	24.0	n/a
Caramel Mini Rolls	Mr Kipling	129	1.6	18.4	5.3	n/a
Caramel Shortcake, each	Mr Kipling	171	1.2	19.9	9.5	n/a
Caramel Supremes	Lyons Bakeries	468	4.9	56.1	24.7	0.3
Caramel Wafers	Tunnock's	454	4.6	68	20.1	n/a
Carbonara Pasta Choice	Crosse & Blackwell	410	18.4	58.4	11.3	2.6
Carbonara Pasta Sauce, chilled	Dolmio	180	3.6	4.6	16.4	n/a
jar	Dolmio	131	1.6	4.5	11.8	n/a
Carbonara Ragu Cream Sauce	Batchelors	152	3.6	2.5	14.2	1.1
Caribbean Chicken Stir Fry	Ross	88.0	5.9	13.8	1.7	1.5

Caribbean Pineapple & Coconut Cooking Sauce	Heinz Weight Watchers	40.0	0.4	6.3	1.5	0.2
Caribbean Prawn Crisps, per pack	Golden Wonder	205	2.7	16.5	14.2	1.7
Carmelle Mix	Green's	117	3.0	17.0	4.0	n/a
Carnation	Nestlé	160	8.2	11.5	9.0	n/a
light	Nestlé	108	7.6	10.5	4.0	n/a
Carnation Slender Plan Drinks						
made with whole milk						
chocolate	Nestlé	229	11.0	27.9	8.2	0.1
coffee	Nestlé	228	11.0	28.4	7.8	Tr
raspberry	Nestlé	228	11.0	28.5	7.8	Tr
strawberry	Nestlé	228	11.0	28.5	7.8	Tr
vanilla	Nestlé	230	11.0	29.0	7.8	Tr
made with semi-skimmed						
chocolate	Nestlé	166	11.3	28.3	0.8	0.1
coffee	Nestlé	165	11.4	28.9	0.4	Tr
raspberry	Nestlé	166	11.4	29.2	0.4	Tr
strawberry	Nestlé	166	11.4	29.2	0.4	Tr
vanilla	Nestlé	167	11.4	29.4	0.4	Tr

Product	*Brand*	*Calories kcal*	*Protein (g)*	*Carbo-hydrate (g)*	*Fat (g)*	*Dietary Fibre (g)*
Carnation Slender Plan Fibre Bars						
apple & banana	Nestlé	385	4.0	63.8	12.6	5.7
apricot	Nestlé	364	5.7	53.4	14.2	11.7
plum	Nestlé	360	4.9	52.9	14.3	9.1
Carrot & Butter Bean Soup	Baxters	47.0	1.6	6.8	1.7	2.3
Carrot & Coriander Reduced Calorie Soup	Batchelors	27.0	1.3	5.2	0.2	n/a
Carrot & Lemon Soup	Baxters	39.0	0.7	6.0	1.5	0.8
Carrot Cake	California Cake & Cookie Ltd	259	2.8	46.8	7.5	1.3
Carrot Juice		24.0	0.5	5.7	0.1	N
Carrot, Onion & Chick Pea Soup	Baxters	34.0	1.7	7.1	0.1	1.5
Carrot, Potato & Coriander Premium Soup	Heinz	34.0	0.7	6.8	0.5	0.8

Carrots						
old, raw		35.0	0.6	7.9	0.3	2.4
old, boiled		24.0	0.6	4.9	0.4	2.5
young, raw		30.0	0.7	6.0	0.5	2.4
young, boiled		22.0	0.6	4.4	0.4	2.3
frozen, boiled		22.0	0.4	4.7	0.3	2.3
canned		20.0	0.5	4.2	0.3	1.9
Cashew Nuts, roasted, salted		611	20.5	18.8	50.9	3.2
	Holland & Barrett	544	17.5	25.0	42.2	11.0
Cashew Pieces	Holland & Barrett	544	17.5	25.0	42.2	11.0
Cassava, fresh, raw		142	0.6	36.8	0.2	1.6
baked		155	0.7	40.1	0.2	1.7
boiled		130	0.5	33.5	0.2	1.4
Casserole Mix	Ross	22.0	0.9	6.2	0.2	1.8
Casserole Mixes (Colman's): *see individual flavours*						
Caster Sugar	Tate & Lyle	400	nil	99.9	nil	nil

All amounts given per 100g/100ml unless otherwise stated

Product	Brand	Calories kcal	Protein (g)	Carbo-hydrate (g)	Fat (g)	Dietary Fibre (g)
Castle Orange Marmalade	Baxters	210	Tr	53.0	nil	0.8
Cauliflower, raw		34.0	3.6	3.0	0.9	1.8
boiled		28.0	2.9	2.1	0.9	1.6
frozen, boiled		20.0	2.0	2.0	0.5	1.2
Cauliflower Cheese		105	5.9	5.1	6.9	1.3
	Heinz Weight Watchers	83.0	5.2	9.6	2.6	0.9
per pack	Birds Eye Menu Master	365	18.0	22.0	23.0	2.7
Cauliflower Cheese Potato Jackets	Birds Eye Country Club	127	5.1	15.4	5.0	0.7
Cauliflower Cheese Quarter Pounders, each	Birds Eye Country Club	220	7.0	17.0	14.0	n/a
Celeriac, raw		18.0	1.2	2.3	0.4	3.7
boiled		15.0	0.9	1.9	0.5	3.2
Celery, raw		7.0	0.5	0.9	0.2	1.1
boiled		8.0	0.5	0.8	0.3	3.2

Channa Masala	Sharwood	120	4.8	10.1	6.7	2.9
Chapati Flour, brown		333	11.5	73.7	1.2	N
white		335	9.8	77.6	0.5	N
Chapati, Paratha & Puri Mix	Sharwood	321	10.2	63.1	2.0	6.6
Chapatis, made with fat		328	8.1	48.3	12.8	N
made without fat		202	7.3	43.7	1.0	N
Chargrill Chicken Mini Bagel, each	Boots Shapers	287	n/a	n/a	n/a	n/a
Chasseur Casserole Recipe Sauce	Knorr	71.0	1.6	10.3	2.9	n/a
Chasseur Cook-In-Sauce Classic	Homepride	47.5	0.8	9.2	0.4	n/a
Cheddar Cheese		412	25.5	0.1	34.4	nil
Cheddar Cheese Crispy Pancakes	Findus	208	7.5	23.0	9.5	0.9
Cheddar Cheese Potatoes 'n' Sauce, as served	Batchelors	459	13.7	70.3	13.9	1.9

Product	Brand	Calories kcal	Protein (g)	Carbo-hydrate (g)	Fat (g)	Dietary Fibre (g)
Cheddar Cheese Slices	Kraft	325	22.0	1.0	26.0	nil
Cheddar-type Cheese, reduced fat		261	31.5	Tr	15.0	nil
Cheddarie Cheddar Cheese Spread	Kraft	280	15.0	8.0	21.0	nil
light	Kraft	240	18.0	8.8	15.0	nil
with Spring Onion	Kraft	275	14.0	7.3	21.0	nil
Cheddars	McVitie's	247	11.0	49.9	32.8	1.9
Cheese: *see individual types*						
Cheese & Chive Golden Lights, per pack	Golden Wonder	98.0	1.1	13.8	4.2	0.7
Cheese & Chives Super-noodles, per packet, as served	Batchelors	522	9.1	65.8	24.7	4.7
Cheese & Ham Dairy Spread, reduced fat	Heinz Weight Watchers	168	16.1	3.5	9.9	nil
Cheese & Ham Pasta Bake Casserole Mix, as sold	Colman's	398	18.0	47.0	15.0	n/a

Cheese & Ham Pasta Rolls	Findus Dinner Supreme	130	7.0	10.3	6.7	0.8
Cheese & Ham Spread, per pack	Boots Shapers	86.0	n/a	n/a	3.1	n/a
Cheese & Herbs Stir & Serve Sauce	Knorr	504	9.0	47.8	30.8	n/a
Cheese & Leek Potatoes 'n' Sauce, as served	Batchelors	455	13.8	70.8	13.1	2.4
Cheese 'n' Onion Cheeselets	Jacob's	480	11.0	58.3	22.5	2.7
Cheese & Onion Crisps, per pack	Golden Wonder	153	2.1	12.5	10.5	1.3
Cheese & Onion Cyborgs	Golden Wonder	89.0	1.3	10.8	4.6	0.3
Cheese & Onion Deep Topped Pizza Slices	McVitie's	223	8.4	30.3	8.2	1.3
Cheese & Onion Pizza, 5"	McCain	168	7.0	29.7	3.2	n/a
Cheese & Onion Sandwich	Jacob's	510	10.3	52.1	28.9	2.3

All amounts given per 100g/100ml unless otherwise stated

Product	*Brand*	*Calories kcal*	*Protein (g)*	*Carbo-hydrate (g)*	*Fat (g)*	*Dietary Fibre (g)*
Cheese & Onion Spread, per pack	Boots Shapers	88.0	n/a	n/a	3.1	n/a
Cheese & Onion Sticks	Jacob's	568	14.2	39.9	39.1	1.5
Cheese & Potato Bake	Tyne Brand	93.0	3.4	10.6	4.1	n/a
Cheese & Tomato Bronto's Monster Feet	McVitie's	240	10.2	33.0	8.1	1.3
Cheese & Tomato French Bread Pizza,	Heinz Weight Watchers	136	10.0	15.1	3.9	2.1
Cheese & Tomato on Sun Dried Tomato Bread Sandwiches, per pack	Boots Shapers	251	n/a	n/a	n/a	n/a
Cheese & Tomato Pizza		235	9.0	24.8	11.8	1.5
	San Marco	244	11.8	24.7	11.3	1.0
5"	McCain	164	6.9	28.3	3.4	n/a
Cheese & Tomato Pizza Rolla	McCain	229	11.7	23.4	10.5	n/a
Cheese & Tomato Sticks	Jacob's	575	14.0	42.0	39.0	1.8

Cheeseburger, each	McDonald's	300	17.0	28.0	13.3	4.0
Cheesecake: ***see also individual flavours***						
Cheesecake, frozen		242	5.7	33.0	10.6	0.9
Cheesecakes	Sunblest	494	4.8	51.4	29.9	1.5
Cheese Dairy Spread, reduced fat	Heinz Weight Watchers	180	16.7	4.2	10.8	nil
Cheese Dry Sauce Mix, as sold	Colman's	389	19.0	46.0	14.0	n/a
Cheese, Leek & Ham Pasta 'n' Sauce	Batchelors	524	23.3	97.8	7.7	9.5
Cheeselet	Jacob's	477	11.2	57.6	22.4	2.7
Cheese, Onion & Chive Dairy Spread, reduced fat	Heinz Weight Watchers	172	15.0	5.5	10.0	0.3
Cheese, Onion & Tomato Lasagne	Birds Eye	128	5.4	12.6	6.2	0.6
Cheese Pour Over Sauce	Baxters	164	5.3	6.3	13.2	0.1

Product	Brand	Calories kcal	Protein (g)	Carbo-hydrate (g)	Fat (g)	Dietary Fibre (g)
Cheese Salad with Plum & Apple Chutney Sandwiches, per pack	Boots Shapers	263	n/a	n/a	n/a	n/a
Cheese Sandwich	Jacob's	514	10.2	52.3	29.3	1.7
Cheese Sauce						
made up with whole milk		197	8.0	9.0	14.6	0.2
with semi-skimmed milk		179	8.1	9.1	12.6	0.2
Cheese Sauce for Lasagne Mix	Knorr	390	17.1	50.8	13.1	n/a
Cheese Sauce Packet Mix						
made up with whole milk		110	5.3	9.3	6.1	N
with semi-skimmed milk		90.0	5.4	9.5	3.8	N
	Knorr	403	16.3	55.3	12.9	n/a
Cheese Spread		276	13.5	4.4	22.8	nil
per pack	Boots Shapers	86.0	n/a	n/a	3.1	n/a
Cheese Spread & Celery, per pack	Boots Shapers	88.0	n/a	n/a	3.1	n/a

Cheese Spread & Chives, per pack	Boots Shapers	87.0	n/a	n/a	3.1	n/a
Cheese Spread, Original, 28g/1oz	Primula	71.0	n/a	n/a	n/a	n/a
with Chives, 28g/1oz	Primula	71.0	n/a	n/a	n/a	n/a
with Ham, 28g/1oz	Primula	71.0	n/a	n/a	n/a	n/a
with Onion, 28g/1oz	Primula	70.0	n/a	n/a	n/a	n/a
with Shrimp, 28g/1oz	Primula	71.0	n/a	n/a	n/a	n/a
Cheese Sticks	Jacob's	569	13.6	38.6	40.0	1.4
Cheese Supreme Deep Pan Pizza	McCain	212	11.0	29.6	6.3	n/a
Cheese, Tomato & Vegetable Deep Crust Pizza Slice	McCain	189	9.3	29.5	4.0	n/a
Cheese, Tomato & Vegetable Pizza Slice	McCain	166	8.9	23.2	4.2	n/a
Cheesey Croquette Royales	Ross	228	4.2	23.7	13.4	1.6
Cheesey Pasta, made up	Kraft	175	4.5	15.4	10.6	0.7

All amounts given per 100g/100ml unless otherwise stated

Product	*Brand*	*Calories kcal*	*Protein (g)*	*Carbo-hydrate (g)*	*Fat (g)*	*Dietary Fibre (g)*
Cheesey Spaghetti	Crosse & Blackwell	69.0	1.9	14.1	0.5	0.5
Cheesey Wotsits, per pack	Golden Wonder	115	2.0	11.8	7.0	n/a
Chelsea Buns		366	7.8	56.1	13.8	1.7
Cherries, raw		48.0	0.9	11.5	0.1	0.9
canned in syrup		71.0	0.5	18.5	Tr	0.6
glacé		251	0.4	66.4	Tr	0.9
Cherryade	Corona	9.0	Tr	10.6	Tr	n/a
Cherry Bakewell	Lyons Bakeries	403	3.8	61.0	15.7	1.1
each	Mr Kipling	206	1.8	31.7	8.0	n/a
Cherry Bio Split Yogurt	Ski	124	4.5	8.3	4.0	nil
Cherry Brandy		255	Tr	32.6	nil	nil
Cherry Cream Cheesecake	McVitie's	336	4.9	30.0	22.0	1.4
Cherry Juice Drink Carton	Robinsons	45.0	Tr	11.0	Tr	n/a
Cherry Pie Filling		82.0	0.4	21.5	Tr	0.4

Cherry Slices, each	Mr Kipling	158	1.5	20.2	7.9	n/a
Cherry Spring, per pack	Boots Shapers	3.0	n/a	n/a	Tr	n/a
Cheshire Cheese		379	24.0	0.1	31.4	nil
Chestnuts		170	2.0	36.6	2.7	4.1
Chewbas, each	Trebor Bassett	14.0	Tr	3.3	0.22	n/a
Chewing Gum: *see individual flavours*						
Chews (Trebor Bassett): *see individual flavours*						
Chicken						
meat only, boiled		183	29.2	nil	7.3	nil
light meat, boiled		163	29.7	nil	4.9	nil
dark meat, boiled		204	28.6	nil	9.9	nil
meat only, roast		148	24.6	nil	5.4	nil
meat & skin, roasted		216	22.6	nil	14.0	nil
light meat, roasted		142	26.5	nil	4.0	nil
dark meat, roasted		155	23.1	nil	6.9	nil
leg quarter, roast, meat only		92.0	15.4	nil	3.4	nil
wing quarter, roast, meat only		74.0	12.4	nil	2.7	nil
breaded, fried in veg. oil		242	18.0	14.8	12.7	0.7

All amounts given per 100g/100ml unless otherwise stated

Product	*Brand*	*Calories kcal*	*Protein (g)*	*Carbo-hydrate (g)*	*Fat (g)*	*Dietary Fibre (g)*
Chicken à La King Simply Fix Dry Mix, as sold	Crosse & Blackwell	420	7.1	41.5	23.8	0.2
Chicken à L'Orange	Findus Lean Cuisine	106	9.0	13.3	1.8	0.8
Chicken & Almond Soup	Baxters	90.0	2.7	4.5	6.8	0.5
Chicken & Bacon Crispy Pancakes	Findus	156	5.7	23.5	4.3	1.0
Chicken & Broccoli Lasagne, per meal	Birds Eye Healthy Options	320	24.0	35.0	9.5	3.2
Chicken & Broccoli Soup	Knorr	337	9.9	60.9	6.0	n/a
Chicken & Garden Vegetables Soup	Knorr	331	10.2	59.3	5.9	n/a
Chicken & Ham Pâté	Shippams	226	15.6	1.3	17.6	n/a
Chicken & Ham with Rice Soup	Heinz Weight Watchers	24.0	1.0	4.2	0.4	0.1
Chicken & Herb Soup	Batchelors	49.0	1.7	3.8	3.1	n/a

Chicken & Leek Cup-A-Soup, per sachet	Batchelors	85.0	1.4	11.5	4.0	n/a
Chicken & Leek Quick Soup	Knorr	496	7.9	45.1	31.5	n/a
Chicken & Leek Slim-A-Soup, per sachet	Batchelors	38.0	1.1	7.9	0.4	n/a
Chicken & Leek Soup	Campbell's	50.0	0.7	3.7	3.5	n/a
Chicken & Mushroom Casserole, per pack	Birds Eye Menu Master	165	18.0	5.0	8.0	0.6
Chicken & Mushroom Crispy Pancake	Findus	191	6.7	24.0	7.6	1.0
Chicken & Mushroom Lasagne Casserole Mix, as sold	Colman's	312	11.0	64.0	1.0	n/a
Chicken & Mushroom Pasta 'n' Sauce, per packet, as served	Batchelors	524	23.1	101	4.7	9.0
Chicken & Mushroom Pot Meal, per pack	Boots Shapers	199	n/a	n/a	4.6	n/a

All amounts given per 100g/100ml unless otherwise stated

Product	*Brand*	*Calories kcal*	*Protein (g)*	*Carbo-hydrate (g)*	*Fat (g)*	*Dietary Fibre (g)*
Chicken & Mushroom Pot Noodle	Golden Wonder	407	13.1	56.0	14.1	n/a
Chicken & Mushroom Slim-A-Soup Special, per sachet	Batchelors	58.0	1.5	8.6	2.2	n/a
Chicken & Mushroom Snack-A-Soup Special, per sachet	Batchelors	187	4.5	26.9	6.8	2.4
Chicken & Mushroom Soup	Campbell's	42.0	0.8	3.1	3.0	n/a
	Heinz	38.0	1.1	3.5	2.2	0.1
Chicken & Mushroom Toast Topper	Heinz	60.0	5.4	6.3	1.5	0.3
Chicken & Prawn Cantonese	Findus Lean Cuisine	102	7.0	10.6	3.4	1.9
Chicken & Sweetcorn Cup-A-Soup Special, per sachet	Batchelors	119	1.4	16.0	5.9	n/a
Chicken & Sweetcorn Pasta Bake Casserole Mix, as sold	Colman's	329	12.0	58.0	5.2	n/a

Chicken & Sweetcorn Soup	Boots Shapers	40.00	n/a	n/a	1.2	n/a
Chicken & Vegetable Cup-A-Soup Special, per sachet	Batchelors	119	1.2	14.1	6.8	n/a
Chicken & Vegetable Masala Potato Topper	Heinz Weight Watchers	68.0	4.8	9.8	1.0	0.8
Chicken & Vegetable Pie	Ross	251	7.3	26.5	13.4	1.1
	Tyne Brand	162	4.7	14.3	9.6	n/a
Chicken & Vegetable Soup	Baxters	31.0	1.3	5.6	0.5	1.6
	Heinz Big Soups	41.0	2.0	6.0	1.0	0.6
Chicken & White Wine Soup	Campbell's	59.0	1.1	3.3	4.7	n/a
Chicken Biryani Microchef Meal	Batchelors	102	7.0	15.3	1.8	n/a
Chicken Breast in Gravy, per pack	Birds Eye Menu Master	165	24.0	4.5	5.5	Tr
Chicken Broth	Baxters	32.0	0.8	5.4	0.9	0.7
Chicken Burgers, each	Birds Eye Steakhouse	160	5.4	12.6	6.2	0.6

All amounts given per 100g/100ml unless otherwise stated

Product	*Brand*	*Calories kcal*	*Protein (g)*	*Carbo-hydrate (g)*	*Fat (g)*	*Dietary Fibre (g)*
Chicken Casserole	Tyne Brand	100	4.2	7.1	6.3	n/a
Chicken Chasseur	Findus Lean Cuisine	95.0	5.7	14.4	1.5	0.6
per meal	Birds Eye Healthy Options	440	27.0	67.0	7.0	2.3
with rice	Heinz Weight Watchers	81.0	4.9	11.2	1.7	0.6
Chicken Chasseur Casserole Mix, as sold	Colman's	284	13.0	54.0	1.2	n/a
Chicken Chasseur Simply Fix Dry Mix, as sold	Crosse & Blackwell	330	11.3	47.9	10.3	1.6
Chicken Cup-A-Noodle, per sachet	Batchelors	138	6.0	27.0	1.1	n/a
Chicken Cup-A-Soup, per sachet	Batchelors	100	1.5	11.5	5.6	n/a
Chicken Curry	Campbell's	87.0	4.9	9.7	3.2	n/a
	Findus Dinner					

	Supreme	127	6.0	18.1	3.4	0.8
	Tyne Brand	149	4.5	11.0	9.7	n/a
with rice	Heinz Lunch Bowl	87.0	3.4	15.7	1.2	0.8
	Heinz Weight Watchers	87.0	4.1	13.4	1.9	0.4
	Vesta	99.0	2.9	20.3	1.2	n/a
per single serving with rice, per pack	Vesta	421	13.0	72.9	8.7	n/a
	Birds Eye Menu Master	430	22.0	63.0	9.5	2.7
Chicken Curry Crispy Pancakes	Findus	168	5.6	23.0	6.0	1.2
Chicken Curry Microchef Meal	Batchelors	143	6.8	21.9	3.1	n/a
Chicken Curry Potato Topper	Heinz	92.0	3.9	9.7	4.2	0.7
Chicken Curry Pot Rice	Golden Wonder	343	11.8	66.7	3.2	n/a
Chicken Fried Rice	Vesta	163	5.9	25.3	4.9	n/a
Chicken Granules, as sold	Oxo	297	13.8	50.8	5.7	n/a

All amounts given per 100g/100ml unless otherwise stated

Product	*Brand*	*Calories kcal*	*Protein (g)*	*Carbo-hydrate (g)*	*Fat (g)*	*Dietary Fibre (g)*
Chicken in Blackbean Sauce	Heinz	100	6.0	16.4	1.2	1.0
Chicken in Curry Mayonnaise Sandwich Maker	Shippams	206	13.1	2.3	16.1	n/a
Chicken in Mayonnaise Sandwich Maker	Shippams	213	13.0	2.3	16.9	n/a
Chicken Korma Bistro Break	HP	117	5.1	15.6	3.0	1.7
Chicken Korma Readymeal	Uncle Ben's	123	9.1	6.3	6.8	n/a
Chicken Korma Simply Fix Dry Mix, as sold	Crosse & Blackwell	430	8.4	49.1	22.2	1.9
Chicken Korma with Pilau Rice	Heinz Weight Watchers	97.0	6.0	11.7	2.9	0.8
Chicken McNuggets (6)	McDonald's	266	18.6	16.9	13.9	1.0
Chicken Marengo with Rice	Heinz Weight Watchers	89.0	6.0	13.4	1.2	0.5
Chicken Masala	Vesta	94.0	3.7	18.1	1.3	n/a

Chicken Noodle & Herb Reduced Calorie Soup	Batchelors	25.0	1.7	4.1	0.2	n/a
Chicken Noodle Soup, dried, as sold		329	13.8	60.9	5.0	4.3
dried, as served		20.0	0.8	3.7	0.3	0.2
Chicken Noodle Soup	Heinz Weight Watchers	18.0	0.9	3.1	0.2	0.1
Chicken Oxo Cubes	Brooke Bond	252	17.3	38.5	4.0	n/a
Chicken Pastini Pasta Soup	Heinz	27.0	1.7	4.0	0.4	0.2
Chicken Pâté	Shippams	233	14.7	1.6	18.6	n/a
Chicken Provençale Simply Fix Dry Mix, as sold	Crosse & Blackwell	360	10.3	53.9	0.7	2.0
Chicken Quick Soup	Knorr	498	7.9	44.9	31.9	n/a
Chicken Ravioli in Tomato Sauce	Heinz	74.0	3.3	13.5	0.4	0.7
Chicken Rice Soup	Campbell's	26.0	0.6	4.4	0.7	n/a
Chicken Risotto, per single serving	Vesta	338	12.4	59.6	5.6	n/a

All amounts given per 100g/100ml unless otherwise stated

Product	*Brand*	*Calories kcal*	*Protein (g)*	*Carbo-hydrate (g)*	*Fat (g)*	*Dietary Fibre (g)*
Chicken Roll with Salad Four Pack Selection Sandwiches, per pack	Boots Shapers	290	n/a	n/a	n/a	n/a
Chicken Savoury Rice, per packet, as served	Batchelors	482	11.9	95.1	6.1	0.6
Chicken Seasoning Dry Sauce Mix, as sold	Colman's	307	11.0	62.0	1.4	n/a
Chicken Slim-A-Soup, per sachet	Batchelors	39.0	1.0	6.8	1.1	n/a
Chicken Soup	Heinz Weight Watchers	22.0	0.8	2.2	1.1	0.1
low calorie	Knorr	303	12.3	61.0	1.1	n/a
Chicken Stew	Campbell's	79.0	4.2	9.8	2.7	n/a
	Tyne Brand	74.0	2.8	5.9	4.4	n/a
Chicken Stock Cubes	Knorr	317	10.2	29.9	17.7	n/a
Chicken Stock Powder	Knorr	210	12.9	28.9	4.8	0.2

Chicken Supernoodles, per packet, as served	Batchelors	519	8.7	66.3	24.5	4.8
Chicken Supreme	Heinz Weight Watchers	89.0	6.0	13.4	1.2	0.5
with rice	Vesta	115	3.6	17.6	3.8	n/a
per pack	Birds Eye Menu Master	413	23.0	56.0	13.0	1.6
per single serving	Vesta	518	17.8	73.6	17.0	n/a
Chicken Supreme Casserole Mix, as sold	Colman's	399	16.0	48.0	15.0	n/a
Chicken Supreme Cook-In-Sauce	Homepride	86.0	1.3	6.9	5.8	n/a
Chicken Sweet & Sour Readymeal	Uncle Ben's	103	6.1	17.5	0.9	n/a
Chicken, Sweetcorn & Asparagus Premium Soup	Heinz	66.0	2.8	5.6	3.5	0.3
Chicken, Sweet Pepper & Dill Premium Soup	Heinz	40.0	1.7	6.2	0.9	0.4

All amounts given per 100g/100ml unless otherwise stated

Product	*Brand*	*Calories kcal*	*Protein (g)*	*Carbo-hydrate (g)*	*Fat (g)*	*Dietary Fibre (g)*
Chicken Tarragon Soup	Campbell's	47.0	1.3	3.8	2.9	n/a
Chicken Tikka & Mayonnaise Pâté	Shippams	273	15.7	4.6	21.3	n/a
Chicken Tikka Masala	Heinz Weight Watchers	94.0	5.7	12.5	2.4	1.1
Chicken Tikka Platter, per meal	Birds Eye Healthy Options	400	30.0	48.0	9.5	3.5
Chicken Tikka with Pilau Rice, per pack	Birds Eye Menu Master	500	26.0	54.0	20.0	3.0
Chicken, Vegetable & Noodle Slim-A-Soup Special, per sachet	Batchelors	55.0	1.7	8.7	1.0	n/a
Chicken with Broccoli Pasta Bake	Heinz Weight Watchers	90.0	6.2	11.1	2.3	0.7
Chick Grills	Ross	324	9.9	21.3	22.5	0.9
Chick Peas						
dried, boiled		121	8.4	18.2	2.1	4.3

canned		115	7.2	16.1	2.9	4.1
	Batchelors	98.0	7.0	21.7	2.2	n/a
Chick Pea Spread: *see Hummus*						
Chicksticks, each	Birds Eye Steakhouse	70.0	3.0	6.5	3.5	0.3
Chicory, raw		11.0	0.5	2.8	0.6	0.9
Chilli & Garlic Sauce	Lea & Perrins	61.0	1.3	12.3	0.7	n/a
Chilli Beanfeast, per packet, as served	Batchelors	389	5.4	65.6	4.6	n/a
Chilli Bean Spread, per pack	Boots Shapers	114	n/a	n/a	4.0	n/a
Chilli Bean Wholesome Soup	Heinz Weight Watchers	33.0	1.7	6.1	0.1	1.2
Chilli Beans		70.0	4.9	12.2	0.5	3.9
	Batchelors	68.0	4.4	12.0	0.3	5.8
Chilli Beef & Bean Spicy Soup	Heinz	36.0	5.6	5.7	0.8	0.8
Chilli Beef & Tomato Snack-A-Soup Special, per sachet	Batchelors	178	4.9	32.1	3.3	2.6

Product	Brand	Calories kcal	Protein (g)	Carbo-hydrate (g)	Fat (g)	Dietary Fibre (g)
Chilli Beef Quarter Pounder, each	Birds Eye Steakhouse	195	15.0	7.0	12.0	1.1
Chilli Con Carne	Campbell's	108	6.2	12.7	3.5	n/a
	Old El Paso	118	9.3	8.3	5.5	n/a
	Tyne Brand	106	9.4	6.6	4.7	n/a
with rice	Heinz Lunch Bowl	98.0	6.4	14.4	1.7	1.9
	Heinz Weight Watchers	88.0	4.8	14.0	1.4	1.0
with rice, per pack	Birds Eye Healthy Options	435	21.0	79.0	4.0	5.0
	Birds Eye Menu Master	403	20.0	63.0	8.0	4.3
Chilli Con Carne Casserole Mix	Colman's	308	8.6	6.2	1.7	n/a
Chilli Con Carne Cook-In-Sauce	Homepride	58.0	2.3	10.6	0.7	n/a
Chilli Con Carne Sauce						

mild	Uncle Ben's	75.0	4.4	13.5	0.6	n/a
medium	Uncle Ben's	79.0	4.5	14.6	0.6	n/a
hot	Uncle Ben's	81.0	4.54	14.8	0.6	n/a
Chilli Con Carne Simply Fix Dry Mix	Crosse & Blackwell	315	12.0	47.7	8.2	3.7
Chilli Con Carne Toast Topper	Heinz	95.0	7.1	9.5	3.2	1.5
Chilli Dip, 28g/1oz	Kavli	98.0	n/a	n/a	n/a	n/a
Chilli Mustard	Colman's	102	6.1	4.1	6.0	n/a
Chilli Peppers						
red, raw		26.0	1.8	4.2	0.3	N
green, raw		20.0	2.9	0.7	0.6	N
Chilli Sauce	Heinz	104	1.4	24.1	0.2	1.1
	HP	128	1.5	28.2	1.0	n/a
Chilli Seasoning Dry Sauce Mix, as sold	Colman's	322	9.2	60.0	3.9	n/a
Chilli with Beans and Vegetables	Tyne Brand	111	5.9	12.5	4.2	n/a

All amounts given per 100g/100ml unless otherwise stated

Product	*Brand*	*Calories kcal*	*Protein (g)*	*Carbo-hydrate (g)*	*Fat (g)*	*Dietary Fibre (g)*
China Fruit Salad in Syrup	Libby	70.0	n/a	n/a	Tr	n/a
Chinese Barbecue Cook-In-Sauce	Homepride	91.0	0.6	21.3	0.1	n/a
Chinese Chicken & Prawn Foo Yeung Stir Fry	Ross	77.0	5.5	12.3	1.4	1.8
Chinese Chicken Flavour Instant Noodles	Sharwood	483	10.2	56.0	17.7	2.3
Chinese Chicken Pot Light	Golden Wonder	323	15.3	62.7	1.3	n/a
Chinese Chicken Soup of the World	Knorr	307	11.1	49.0	7.4	n/a
Chinese Chicken Stir Fry	Ross	57.0	5.7	9.6	0.8	2.8
Chinese Chow Mein Super-noodles, per packet, as served	Batchelors	519	8.7	65.9	24.5	4.7
Chinese Curry Flavour Instant Noodles	Sharwood	442	9.8	55.8	19.2	3.1

Chinese Mushroom, dried		284	10.0	59.9	1.8	Tr
Chinese Noodle Quick Serve Soup, as served	Batchelors	121	4.2	23.7	1.3	n/a
Chinese Oxo Cubes, each, as sold	Brooke Bond	18.0	0.6	2.9	0.5	n/a
Chinese Pouring Sauces (Sharwood): ***see individual flavours***						
Chinese Prawns Stir Fry	Ross	60.0	3.3	12.4	0.4	1.5
Chinese Sauce Mixes (Sharwood): ***see individual flavours***						
Chinese Sizzling Prawns Stir Fry	Ross	39.0	3.3	8.2	0.3	2.5
Chinese Special Fried Savoury Rice, per packet, as served	Batchelors	440	11.3	97.0	4.1	5.6
Chinese Special Rice	Ross	99.0	4.1	21.1	0.3	1.0
Chinese Spring Rolls	Ross	114	4.0	22.5	1.6	1.7
Chinese Style Beanfeast, per packet, as served	Batchelors	287	22.6	65.6	4.6	n/a

Product	*Brand*	*Calories kcal*	*Protein (g)*	*Carbo-hydrate (g)*	*Fat (g)*	*Dietary Fibre (g)*
Chinese Sweet & Sour Pork Stir Fry	Ross	63.0	4.1	12.0	0.8	2.1
Chinese Sweet & Sour Sauce	Campbell's	70.0	0.4	16.4	0.3	n/a
Chinese Szechuan Cooking Sauce	Heinz Weight Watchers	42.0	1.0	5.9	1.7	0.7
Chinese Tomato & Noodle Instant Soup, as sold	Knorr	348	6.3	66.4	8.2	4.0
Chips						
crinkle cut, frozen, fried		290	3.6	33.4	16.7	2.2
French fries, retail		280	3.3	34.0	15.5	2.1
homemade, fried		189	3.9	30.1	6.7	2.2
retail		239	3.2	30.5	12.4	2.2
straight cut, frozen, fried		273	4.1	36.0	13.5	2.4
Chips, microwave		221	3.6	32.1	9.6	2.9
Chips, oven		162	3.2	29.8	4.2	2.0
Chip Shop Battered Fish						

Cakes	Ross	232	10.6	19.7	12.7	0.8
Chip Shop Chips	Ross	75.0	2.0	17.6	0.2	1.3
Chip Shop Fish Cakes	Ross	232	10.6	19.7	12.7	0.8
Chip Shop Jumbo Cod & Chips	Ross	169	6.1	19.1	7.9	0.8
Chip Shop Jumbo Cod Fish Fingers	Ross	232	10.2	14.2	15.2	0.7
Chip Shop Jumbo Cod Steaks	Ross	180	10.4	11.5	10.5	0.5
Chip Shop Jumbo Fish Steaks	Ross	186	11.0	13.9	9.9	0.6
Chip Shop Mushy Peas	Ross	117	7.5	23.0	0.2	1.8
Chip Shop Scampi	Ross	228	8.3	22.8	11.9	1.0
Chip Shop Scampi Fries	Ross	228	8.3	22.8	11.9	0.9
Choc Chip & Hazelnut Cookies	McVitie's	504	5.4	65.2	24.3	2.0
Choc Chip & Orange Cookies	McVitie's	501	5.3	65.8	23.8	2.0

All amounts given per 100g/100ml unless otherwise stated

Product	Brand	Calories kcal	Protein (g)	Carbo-hydrate (g)	Fat (g)	Dietary Fibre (g)
Choc Chip Harvest Chewy Bar, each	Quaker	112	1.5	17.3	4.0	0.8
Choc Chip Tracker	Mars	504	9.1	56.3	26.9	n/a
Chocaholics Dessert	Chambourcy	230	4.5	23.7	13.2	0.4
Chococino Hot Chcolate Drink, as sold	Nestlé	437	12.3	61.0	16.0	0.6
Chococino Lite, as sold	Nestlé	359	18.0	54.9	7.5	2.9
Chocolate: *see individual flavours*						
Chocolate & Caramel Bar, per pack	Boots Shapers	97.0	n/a	n/a	4.9	n/a
Chocolate & Orange Royale	McVitie's	286	5.6	27.5	17.1	0.2
Chocolate & Vanilla Rolls	Lyons Bakeries	448	3.7	53.2	24.3	0.7
Chocolate Bar Cake	McVitie's	377	4.8	53.8	14.9	1.3
Chocolate Biscuits, full-coated		524	5.7	67.4	27.6	2.1
Chocolate Blancmange						

Powder, as sold	Brown & Polson	339	2.7	78.0	1.7	n/a
Chocolate Buttons	Cadbury	525	7.8	56.8	29.4	n/a
Chocolate Cake	Cadbury	384	4.7	58.1	14.2	n/a
Chocolate Chip Cake Bars, each	Mr Kipling	126	1.5	13.2	7.1	n/a
Chocolate Chip Cookies	Cadbury	485	6.4	68.3	20.7	1.7
	California Cake & Cookie Ltd	452	4.7	59.7	23.2	0.8
Chocolate Chip Muffin	California Cake & Cookie Ltd	330	5.8	44.9	15.3	0.9
Chocolate Chip Solar	McVitie's	472	6.7	56.8	24.1	2.2
Chocolate Cream	Cadbury	430	2.7	69.6	14.7	n/a
Chocolate Creme de Creme, each	Lyons Maid	161	3.2	17.5	8.8	n/a
Chocolate Crusha	Burgess	166	nil	41.5	nil	nil
Chocolate Cup Cakes	Lyons Bakeries	344	2.4	74.3	4.1	0.6

All amounts given per 100g/100ml unless otherwise stated

Product	*Brand*	*Calories kcal*	*Protein (g)*	*Carbo-hydrate (g)*	*Fat (g)*	*Dietary Fibre (g)*
Chocolate Digestive Bars	McVitie's	513	6.5	63.0	26.0	2.2
Chocolate Digestive Biscuit	Holland & Barrett	487	5.2	63.7	23.6	nil
Chocolate Digestives: *see Digestive Biscuits*						
Chocolate Eclairs	Cravens	479	2.8	71.9	20.1	0.5
Chocolate Fancies	Lyons Bakeries	511	5.3	55.8	29.6	0.3
Chocolate Farls	Tunnock's	521	5.5	62.8	27.5	n/a
Chocolate Flavour Rice	Ambrosia	106	3.5	16.9	2.8	n/a
Chocolate Fondant Fancies, each	Mr Kipling	111	0.8	19.9	3.2	n/a
Chocolate Fruit & Nut Crunch	Mornflake	400	12.0	60.0	12.5	6.5
Chocolate Fudge Slices, each	Mr Kipling	152	1.1	20.2	7.0	n/a
Chocolate Hazlenut Club Class	Jacob's	521	6.5	56.7	29.8	2.5
Chocolate Hob Nobs	McVitie's	497	6.3	62.8	24.3	3.7

Chocolate Homewheat	McVitie's	507	6.5	64.8	24.3	2.5
Chocolate Ice Cream	Fiesta	187	3.5	20.6	10.6	n/a
	Lyons Maid	91.0	2.0	11.4	4.2	n/a
per pack	Boots Shapers	130	n/a	n/a	5.5	n/a
Chocolate Jaspers	McVitie's	506	6.0	64.7	24.5	2.7
Chocolate Limes	Cravens	406	0.6	90.9	4.5	0.3
Chocolate M & Ms	Mars	480	6.0	68.2	20.4	n/a
Chocolate Microbake Sponge Pudding	Homepride	307	6.0	51.0	9.0	n/a
Chocolate Mini Rolls, each	Cadbury	119	1.4	15.6	5.5	n/a
Chocolate Mint Creams, each	Trebor Bassett	39.0	0.1	7.8	0.8	nil
Chocolate Mint Crisp	Cravens	408	0.7	90.4	9.4	0.4
Chocolate Mousse		139	4.0	19.9	5.4	N
each	Fiesta	83.0	1.9	10.2	3.8	n/a

All amounts given per 100g/100ml unless otherwise stated

Product	*Brand*	*Calories kcal*	*Protein (g)*	*Carbo-hydrate (g)*	*Fat (g)*	*Dietary Fibre (g)*
Chocolate Nesquik	Nestlé	371	3.1	83.4	2.8	0.8
made up with whole milk	Nestlé	171	7.1	18.5	8.1	0.1
with semi-skimmed milk	Nestlé	134	7.1	18.5	4.0	0.1
ready to drink	Nestlé	90.0	3.3	11.3	3.5	Tr
Chocolate Nut Spread		549	6.0	60.5	33.0	0.8
Chocolate Nut Sundae		278	3.0	34.2	15.3	0.1
Chocolate Oliver Biscuits	Fortts	359	6.5	69.5	23.9	3.9
Chocolate Perkin	Tunnock's	506	7.5	62.0	25.9	n/a
Chocolate Ready Brek	Weetabix	377	10.5	61.9	9.7	8.4
Chocolate Ripple Dairy Ice Cream	Heinz Weight Watchers	137	3.2	18.7	5.0	0.4
Chocolate Ripple Ice Cream	Lyons Maid	98.0	2.0	14.2	3.7	n/a
Chocolate Ripple Napoli	Lyons Maid	121	2.3	14.9	5.9	n/a
Chocolate Roll	Cadbury	418	5.0	56.3	17.3	n/a

Chocolate Sandwich	Lyons Bakeries	377	4.5	51.8	16.6	0.9
Chocolate Sundae, per pack	Boots Shapers	146	n/a	n/a	5.8	n/a
Chocolate Swiss Roll	Mr Kipling	328	4.3	53.0	12.5	n/a
Chocolate Swiss Rolls	Lyons Bakeries	390	4.8	55.7	16.4	1.3
Chocolate Trifle	St Ivel	247	4.1	23.2	15.9	n/a
per pack	Boots Shapers	117	n/a	n/a	4.9	n/a
Chocolate Truffle Cheesecake	McVitie's	340	5.9	35.4	19.7	0.6
Chocolate with Chocolate Sauce Sponge Pudding	Heinz	288	2.8	47.6	9.6	1.5
Chocolate with Orange Liqueur Dessert Bombes	Heinz Weight Watchers	128	2:3	24.0	2.4	6.2
Chocolova	McVitie's	351	3.4	42.3	18.7	Tr
Choicegrain Cracker	Jacob's	436	8.9	66.7	14.8	3.5
Choice Wholemeal Biscuits	McVitie's	481	7.6	66.5	19.9	6.5
Chomp	Cadbury	460	4.4	67.5	19.4	n/a

All amounts given per 100g/100ml unless otherwise stated

Product	Brand	Calories kcal	Protein (g)	Carbo-hydrate (g)	Fat (g)	Dietary Fibre (g)
Chopped Ham & Pork, canned		275	14.4	1.4	23.6	0.3
Chopped Tomatoes	Napolina	15.0	1.2	2.5	Tr	n/a
for Bolognese	Napolina	24.0	1.4	5.0	Tr	n/a
with Herbs	Napolina	14.0	1.2	2.5	Tr	n/a
with Onions & Herbs	Napolina	16.0	1.2	3.0	Tr	n/a
Chop Suey Stir Fry Sauce	Homepride	53.0	0.5	11.3	0.7	n/a
	Sharwood	75.0	0.7	14.6	1.5	0.2
Chow Mein	Vesta	105	4.6	18.5	1.9	n/a
per single serving	Vesta	337	13.5	58.6	5.4	n/a
Chow Mein Microchef Snack	Batchelors	63.0	4.1	11.1	0.6	n/a
Chow Mein Mix	Ross	58.0	2.2	13.3	0.4	1.8
Chow Mein Pot Noodle	Golden Wonder	398	13.4	59.0	12.0	n/a
Christmas Cake	Mr Kipling	359	3.1	64.7	8.1	n/a
Christmas Log	Mr Kipling	436	4.9	57.0	19.2	n/a
Christmas Mince Pies, each	Mr Kipling	253	2.4	40.3	9.1	n/a

Christmas Pudding, recipe		291	4.6	49.5	9.7	1.3
retail		329	3.0	56.3	11.8	1.7
Christmas Slices, each	Mr Kipling	192	1.1	36.8	3.7	n/a
Chunky Aero	Nestlé	530	8.2	54.2	31.1	n/a
Chunky Chicken Curry	Shippams	121	12.0	4.6	6.2	n/a
Chunky Chicken Supreme	Shippams	159	13.0	4.5	10.1	n/a
Chunky Chips	Ross	118	2.4	21.9	3.0	1.6
Chutney: ***see individual flavours***						
Cider, dry		36.0	Tr	2.6	nil	nil
sweet		42.0	Tr	4.3	nil	nil
vintage		101	Tr	7.3	nil	nil
low alcohol	Strongbow	16.0	n/a	n/a	n/a	n/a
Cider Apple with Herbs Stuffing Mix	Knorr	417	10.0	64.7	13.1	n/a
Cider Vinegar	Holland & Barrett	1.8	nil	0.4	nil	0.4

All amounts given per 100g/100ml unless otherwise stated

Product	Brand	Calories kcal	Protein (g)	Carbo-hydrate (g)	Fat (g)	Dietary Fibre (g)
Citrus Fruit Drink	Rowntree	48.0	Tr	11.7	Tr	nil
per pack	Boots Shapers	nil	n/a	n/a	nil	n/a
Classic Bean Salad	Batchelors	98.0	5.7	19.8	1.1	3.6
Classic Chinese Marinade	Sharwood	115	1.8	16.1	4.8	1.0
Classic Chocolate Cake	Lyons Bakeries	466	6.4	50.9	26.2	0.6
Classic Chocolate Roll	Lyons Bakeries	420	4.8	55.0	20.1	0.6
Classic French Vinaigrette Maker	Lea & Perrins	117	1.3	24.3	1.5	n/a
Clear Country Vegetable Soup	Knorr	291	6.3	59.8	2.9	n/a
Clementines, flesh only		37	0.9	8.7	0.1	1.2
Clementines in Natural Juice	Libby	41.0	n/a	n/a	Tr	n/a
Cloudy Lemonade, per pack	Boots Shapers	nil	n/a	n/a	nil	n/a
Clover	Dairy Crest	388	7.1	n/a	39.9	n/a
Club Biscuits (Jacob's): *see individual flavours*						

Coca-Cola		39.0	Tr	10.5	nil	nil
Cock-a-Leekie Soup	Baxters	22.0	0.5	3.9	0.6	0.5
Cockles, boiled		48.0	17.2	Tr	2.0	nil
Cocktail Cherries	Burgess	247	0.3	61.4	nil	0.9
Cocktail Dressing For Seafood & Salads	Crosse & Blackwell	146	1.0	14.4	8.9	0.3
Cocktail Sausage Rolls	Kraft	320	6.6	24.7	22.3	n/a
Cocoa Powder		312	18.5	11.5	21.7	12.1
made up with whole milk		76.0	3.4	6.8	4.2	0.2
made up with semi-skimmed milk		57.0	3.5	7.0	1.9	0.2
Coconut, creamed		669	6.0	7.0	68.8	N
desiccated		604	5.6	6.4	62.0	13.7
Coconut & Pineapple Yogurt Mousse, per pack	Boots Shapers	80.0	n/a	n/a	3.7	n/a
Coconut Bar, each	Boots Shapers	97.0	n/a	n/a	3.7	n/a
Coconut Crumble	Jacob's	505	5.4	56.0	28.0	5.9

All amounts given per 100g/100ml unless otherwise stated

Product	Brand	Calories kcal	Protein (g)	Carbo-hydrate (g)	Fat (g)	Dietary Fibre (g)
Coconut Hot Chocolate, per pack	Boots Shapers	40.0	n/a	n/a	0.9	n/a
Coconut Macaroons, each	Mr Kipling	117	0.9	16.4	5.3	n/a
Coconut Oil		899	Tr	nil	99.9	nil
Coco Pops	Kellogg's	380	5.0	87.0	0.8	1.0
Cod, dried, salted, boiled		138	32.5	nil	0.9	nil
Cod & Prawn Pie	Ross	164	8.7	11.9	9.3	0.5
Cod Crumble	Ross	179	8.9	12.7	10.5	0.5
Cod Fillet Fish Cakes in Crispy Crunch Crumb, each	Birds Eye Captain's Table	85.0	4.5	8.5	3.5	0.3
Cod Fillet Fish Fingers grilled, each	Ross Birds Eye Captain's Table Findus	182 50.0 205	11.5 3.5 12.0	17.4 5.0 16.5	8.7 2.0 10.0	0.7 0.2 0.2

Cod Fillets

baked		96.0	21.4	nil	1.2	nil
poached		94.0	20.9	nil	1.1	nil
in Natural Crumb	Ross	180	11.1	17.9	7.4	0.8
Cod Fillet Steaks in Battercrisp	Findus	208	11.2	13.7	12.1	0.5
Cod Fillet Steaks in Light Crispy Crumb	Findus	215	12.6	16.7	11.2	0.6
Cod Fish Fingers	Ross	182	11.5	17.4	8.7	0.7
each	Birds Eye					
	Captain's Table	45.0	3.0	2.0	4.0	n/a
Cod Liver Oil		899	Tr	nil	99.9	nil
Cod Mornay, per pack	Birds Eye Menu Master	415	29.0	23.0	23.0	0.3
Cod Roe, hard, fried		202	20.9	3.0	11.9	0.1
Cod Steak in Butter Sauce	Findus	108	10.9	3.8	5.5	Tr
	Ross	84.0	10.5	3.0	3.4	0.1
per pack	Birds Eye					
	Captain's Table	119	18.0	9.0	9.5	0.1

All amounts given per 100g/100ml unless otherwise stated

Product	*Brand*	*Calories kcal*	*Protein (g)*	*Carbo-hydrate (g)*	*Fat (g)*	*Dietary Fibre (g)*
Cod Steak in Cheese Sauce, per pack	Birds Eye Captain's Table	175	20.0	9.5	6.5	0.1
Cod Steak in Mushroom Sauce, per pack	Birds Eye Captain's Table	168	18.0	9.0	8.0	0.2
Cod Steak in Parsley Sauce per pack	Ross	89.0	10.4	2.9	4.0	0.1
	Birds Eye Captain's Table	170	19.0	11.0	5.5	0.2
	Findus	104	10.6	3.7	5.2	Tr
Cod Steaks						
grilled		95.0	20.8	nil	1.3	nil
in batter, fried in oil		199	19.6	nil	10.3	0.3
Cod Steaks in Crispy Crunch Crumb, each	Birds Eye Captain's Table	225	14.0	13.0	13.0	0.9
Cod Steaks in Harvest Crumb, each	Birds Eye Captain's Table	185	13.0	13.0	19.0	1.8
Cod Steaks in Natural Crumb	Ross	180	11.1	17.9	7.4	0.8

Cod Steaks in Waferlight Batter, each	Birds Eye Captain's Table	225	12.0	15.0	13.0	0.5
Coffee, infusion, 5 minutes		2.0	0.2	0.3	Tr	nil
instant		100	14.6	11.0	Tr	nil
Coffee Matchmakers	Nestlé	474	5.0	65.3	21.4	n/a
Coffee-Mate, per 4.5g tsp						
regular	Carnation	25.0	0.1	2.5	1.6	nil
lite	Carnation	19.0	Tr	3.0	0.7	nil
Coffee Napoli	Lyons Maid	98.0	1.9	10.4	5.5	n/a
Coffee Walnut Whip	Nestlé	490	5.8	60.3	25.1	n/a
Cola Refresher, each	Trebor Bassett	7.6	nil	1.4	nil	nil
Coleslaw	Heinz	134	1.4	9.5	10.1	1.0
	St Ivel Shape	95.0	1.7	5.5	7.4	1.6
Coley Fillet, steamed		99.0	23.3	nil	0.6	nil
Common Sense Oat Bran Flakes	Kellogg's	360	12.0	65.0	5.0	10.0

All amounts given per 100g/100ml unless otherwise stated

Product	*Brand*	*Calories kcal*	*Protein (g)*	*Carbo-hydrate (g)*	*Fat (g)*	*Dietary Fibre (g)*
Common Sense Oat Bran Flakes with Raison & Apple	Kellogg's	340	11.0	65.0	4.5	9.0
Complete Custard Mix	Rowntree	412	4.2	27.8	10.2	n/a
Compound Cooking Fat		894	Tr	Tr	99.3	nil
Condensed Milk						
sweetened, skimmed		267	10.0	60.0	0.2	nil
sweetened, whole		333	8.5	55.5	10.1	nil
Conservation Grade Porridge Oats	Jordans	379	12.0	66.0	7.4	7.0
Consomme	Campbell's	7.0	1.2	0.5	nil	nil
	Crosse & Blackwell	20.0	4.0	0.9	Tr	Tr
Continental Mix	Ross	37.0	1.6	8.9	0.4	2.2
Continental Style Wholemeal Loaf	Holland & Barrett	218	10.0	41.4	2.4	8.8
Contrast	Cadbury	475	4.2	62.1	23.6	n/a

Cookeen Cooking fat	Van Den Berghs	900	nil	nil	100	nil
Cookies & Cream Premium Ice Cream	Heinz Weight Watchers	175	3.5	23.9	6.8	nil
Cooking Mixes and Sauces (Colman's): ***see individual flavours***						
Coolmints, each	Trebor Bassett	3.7	nil	1.5	nil	nil
Coq au Vin	Baxters	77.0	10.5	3.2	2.6	0.4
Coq au Vin Casserole Mix, as sold	Colman's	292	7.7	60.0	1.5	n/a
Corned Beef, canned		217	26.9	nil	26.9	nil
	Libby	224	24.5	1.0	13.5	nil
Corn Flakes	Kellogg's	370	7.0	83.0	0.7	1.0
	Sunblest	377	8.1	84.0	1.0	1.6
Cornflour		354	0.6	92.0	0.7	0.1
Cornish Ice Cream	Lyons Maid	92.0	19.	11.3	4.4	n/a
Cornish Pastie		332	8.0	31.1	20.4	0.9
Cornish Wafers	Jacob's	530	8.3	54.0	31.2	2.3

Product	Brand	Calories kcal	Protein (g)	Carbo-hydrate (g)	Fat (g)	Dietary Fibre (g)
Corn Oil	Mazola	900	Tr	nil	99.9	n/a
Corn on the Cob, whole, raw		54.0	2.0	9.9	1.0	0.9
boiled		66.0	2.5	11.6	1.4	1.3
Corn Pops	Kellogg's	380	5.0	88.0	1.5	1.0
Coronation Sauce	Heinz	334	0.8	13.1	3.9	0.9
Cottage Cheese						
plain		98.0	13.8	2.1	3.9	nil
	St Ivel Shape	67.0	10.8	5.5	0.2	nil
with additions		95.0	12.8	2.6	3.8	Tr
reduced fat		78.0	13.3	3.3	1.4	Tr
Cottage Pie	Findus Lean Cuisine	93.0	5.0	11.8	2.9	0.7
Cough Candy	Cravens	386	Tr	96.4	nil	nil
Cough Candy Twists, each	Trebor Bassett	27.8	nil	6.9	nil	nil
Country Bean with Mushroom Premium Soup	Heinz	56.0	2.9	8.0	1.4	1.6

Country Beef Recipe Sauce, dry, as sold	Knorr	319	9.6	58.0	7.0	4.2
Country Chicken Recipe Sauce, dry, as sold	Knorr	352	4.4	58.4	12.8	3.8
Country French Chicken Tonight Sauce	Batchelors	117	0.7	6.6	9.7	n/a
Country French Chicken Tonight Sauce	Batchelors	117	0.7	6.6	9.7	n/a
Country Fruit Cake	Mr Kipling	378	4.7	54.1	15.3	n/a
Country Fruit Cake Bars, each	Mr Kipling	120	1.2	17.0	5.1	n/a
Country Fruit Lemon Tart	Mr Kipling	401	4.1	60.6	15.7	n/a
Country Garden Soup	Baxters	28.0	0.7	5.4	0.5	0.8
Country Grain Multigrain Wholemeal Bread	Hovis	216	10.4	37.1	2.9	7.1
Country Mix Vegetables	Ross	31.0	2.1	6.8	0.5	2.4
Country Oatmeal Crunch Biscuits	Peek Frean	457	6.9	66.8	18.0	3.6

All amounts given per 100g/100ml unless otherwise stated

Product	*Brand*	*Calories kcal*	*Protein (g)*	*Carbo-hydrate (g)*	*Fat (g)*	*Dietary Fibre (g)*
Country Slices, each	Mr Kipling	126	1.5	19.0	4.9	n/a
Country Store	Kellogg's	360	9.0	69.0	5.0	7.0
Country Style Chicken Casserole Recipe Sauce	Knorr	34.0	0.8	8.0	0.1	n/a
Country Style Chunky Chicken	Shippams	171	13.0	3.9	11.9	n/a
Country Tomato & Bean Wholesoup, as served	Batchelors	325	15.8	68.0	3.5	10.3
Country Tomato Reduced Calorie Soup	Batchelors	27.0	1.6	4.1	0.4	n/a
Country Tomato Soup	Batchelors	60.0	1.4	6.3	3.3	n/a
Country Vegetable & Beef Soup	Heinz Weight Watchers	26.0	1.2	4.8	0.3	0.5
Country Vegetable Soup	Heinz Weight Watchers	24.0	0.8	4.8	0.2	0.7
Courgettes (zucchini, squash), raw		18.0	1.8	1.8	0.4	0.9

boiled		19.0	2.0	2.0	0.4	1.2
fried in corn oil		63.0	2.6	2.6	4.8	1.2
Crab, boiled		127	20.1	nil	5.2	nil
canned		81.0	18.1	nil	0.9	nil
Crab Pâté	Shippams	96.0	15.9	1.2	3.1	n/a
Cracker Barrel Cheddar Cheese	Kraft	410	26.0	0.1	34.0	nil
Crackerbread	Ryvita	376	0.9	71.3	2.5	2.9
with high fibre	Ryvita	304	3.8	56.9	2.3	18.3
Cranberry & Orange Sauce	Colman's	274	0.2	67.0	0.2	n/a
Cranberry Jelly	Baxters	255	Tr	68.0	Tr	1.7
Cranberry Sauce	Baxters	126	0.1	33.3	nil	1.4
	Burgess	205	nil	50.7	nil	1.2
Cream, fresh (pasteurised)						
clotted		586	1.6	2.3	63.5	nil
double		449	1.7	2.7	48.0	nil
half		148	3.0	4.3	13.3	nil

All amounts given per 100g/100ml unless otherwise stated

Product	Brand	Calories kcal	Protein (g)	Carbo-hydrate (g)	Fat (g)	Dietary Fibre (g)
single		198	2.6	4.1	19.1	nil
soured		205	2.9	3.8	19.9	nil
whipping		373	2.0	3.1	39.3	nil
Cream, sterilised, canned		239	2.5	3.7	23.9	nil
Cream, UHT, aerosol spray		309	1.9	3.5	32.0	nil
Cream Cheese		439	3.1	Tr	47.4	nil
Cream Crackers		440	9.5	68.3	16.3	2.2
	Jacob's	444	10.0	68.0	14.7	2.3
Creamed Garlic Sauce	Burgess	424	2.5	20.3	36.1	1.5
Creamed Horseradish	Burgess	197	2.6	21.7	10.2	2.1
	Colman's	229	4.3	21.0	13.0	n/a
Creamed Macaroni	Ambrosia	90.0	4.0	14.6	1.7	n/a
Creamed Rice	Ambrosia	90.0	3.4	15.2	1.6	n/a
low fat	Ambrosia	76.0	3.6	13.6	0.8	n/a
Creamed Rice Pudding	Libby	88.0	3.2	15.2	1.6	0.2

Creamed Rice Pudding Dessert Pots	Ambrosia	99.0	3.4	16.4	2.2	n/a
Creamed Sago	Ambrosia	80.0	2.9	13.5	1.6	n/a
Creamed Semolina	Ambrosia	82.0	3.6	13.2	1.7	n/a
Creamed Tapioca	Ambrosia	81.0	2.9	13.8	1.6	n/a
Creamed Tomato Soup	Crosse & Blackwell	76.0	0.7	10.0	3.7	0.1
Cream of Asparagus Cup-A-Soup Special, per sachet	Batchelors	127	1.1	17.1	6.5	n/a
Cream of Asparagus Soup	Baxters	66.0	0.9	4.8	4.9	0.2
	Campbell's	43.0	3.2	4.0	2.7	n/a
	Heinz	43.0	0.9	3.6	2.8	0.2
Cream of Asparagus Stir & Serve Soup	Knorr	520	6.3	45.0	35.0	n/a
Cream of Broccoli Stir & Serve Soup	Knorr	513	6.6	46.1	33.6	n/a
Cream of Celery Soup	Campbell's	47.0	0.7	3.1	3.5	n/a
	Heinz	43.0	0.9	3.6	2.8	0.2

All amounts given per 100g/100ml unless otherwise stated

Product	Brand	Calories kcal	Protein (g)	Carbo-hydrate (g)	Fat (g)	Dietary Fibre (g)
Cream of Celery Stir & Serve Soup	Knorr	507	6.4	42.8	34.5	n/a
Cream of Chicken & Mushroom Stir & Serve Soup	Knorr	520	6.9	44.4	35.0	n/a
Cream of Chicken Packet Soup, as served	Batchelors	458	10.6	54.2	23.4	3.2
Cream of Chicken Quick Serve Soup, as served	Batchelors	338	5.0	39.5	18.4	n/a
Cream of Chicken Soup,						
canned, ready to serve		58.0	1.7	4.5	3.8	N
condensed, ready to serve		98.0	2.6	6.0	7.2	N
	Campbell's	50.0	1.0	3.7	3.5	n/a
	Crosse & Blackwell	59.0	1.0	4.7	4.0	Tr
	Heinz	48.0	1.2	4.0	3.1	0.1
	Knorr	377	10.5	59.0	11.0	n/a
Cream of Garden Veg. Packet						

Soup, as served	Batchelors	474	10.5	68.4	20.2	5.9
Cream of Herb Packet Serve Soup, as served	Batchelors	281	2.1	34.4	15.5	n/a
Cream of Herb Soup	Batchelors	43.0	1.6	1.5	3.5	n/a
Cream of Leek Soup	Baxters	45.0	0.6	5.8	2.4	0.4
Cream of Leek Stir & Serve Soup	Knorr	509	5.4	46.4	33.5	n/a
Cream of Mushroom Packet Soup, as served	Batchelors	497	5.7	62.3	26.2	2.9
Cream of Mushroom Soup, canned, ready to serve		53	1.1	3.9	3.8	N
	Campbell's	49.0	0.7	3.5	3.6	n/a
	Crosse & Blackwell	59.0	0.8	5.0	3.9	0.2
	Knorr	462	8.6	48.8	25.8	n/a
Cream of Mushroom Stir & Serve Soup	Knorr	519	4.4	45.3	35.6	n/a

All amounts given per 100g/100ml unless otherwise stated

Product	*Brand*	*Calories kcal*	*Protein (g)*	*Carbo-hydrate (g)*	*Fat (g)*	*Dietary Fibre (g)*
Cream of Onion Soup	Campbell's	44.0	0.5	4.0	2.8	n/a
Cream of Prawn Soup	Campbell's	540	1.2	4.2	3.6	n/a
Cream of Tomato Quick Serve Soup, as served	Batchelors	359	2.9	55.8	14.5	n/a
Cream of Tomato Soup						
canned, ready to serve		55.0	0.8	5.9	3.3	N
condensed, ready to serve		123	1.7	14.6	6.8	N
	Baxters	69.0	1.1	10.3	2.9	0.3
	Heinz	57.0	0.8	7.3	2.8	0.7
	Knorr	448	3.0	58.8	22.3	n/a
Cream of Vegetable Cup-A-Soup Special, per sachet	Batchelors	120	1.7	15.3	6.2	n/a
Cream of Vegetable Stir & Serve Soup	Knorr	460	6.4	42.5	29.4	n/a
Cream Rock, each	Trebor Bassett	14.0	Tr	3.4	0.1	Tr
Cream Soda	Barr	29.0	Tr	7.2	Tr	Tr
	Idris	20.0	nil	5.2	nil	n/a

Cream Toffee Assorted, each	Trebor Bassett	37.5	0.2	5.5	1.5	nil
Cream Toffee Liquorice, each	Trebor Bassett	36.4	0.2	5.6	1.4	nil
Creamy Chicken Pot Rice	Golden Wonder	355	12.6	68.2	3.5	n/a
Creamy Curry Chicken Tonight Sauce	Batchelors	102	1.2	5.7	8.3	n/a
Creamy Curry Low In Fat Sauce	Homepride	310	1.4	8.4	3.9	n/a
Creamy Highland Veg. Soup	Baxters	56.0	1.1	7.2	2.7	1.1
Creamy Mushroom Chicken Tonight Sauce	Batchelors	97.0	0.6	5.2	8.2	n/a
Creamy Mushroom Stir & Serve Sauce	Knorr	521	8.2	43.8	34.8	n/a
Creamy Tomato & Mushroom Pasta 'n' Sauce, as served	Batchelors	461	22.9	79.4	6.0	9.6

All amounts given per 100g/100ml unless otherwise stated

Product	Brand	Calories kcal	Protein (g)	Carbo-hydrate (g)	Fat (g)	Dietary Fibre (g)
Creamy White Sauce, as sold	Oxo	447	4.9	60.3	20.7	n/a
Creme Caramel		109	3.0	20.6	2.2	N
	Chambourcy	110	3.8	20.3	1.5	nil
	St Ivel	104	3.4	20.0	1.2	0.2
Creme Eggs		385	4.1	58.0	16.8	Tr
Creole Chicken Deep South Recipe	Homepride	78.0	1.5	13.7	2.1	n/a
Crinkle Cut Chips	McCain	131	2.6	21.0	4.1	n/a
Crinkle Microchips	McCain	187	2.5	27.4	8.2	n/a
Crinkles Oven Chips	McCain	157	1.9	26.7	4.7	n/a
Crisps: *see individual flavours*						
Crispy Caramel, each	Boots Shapers	97.0	n/a	n/a	4.4	n/a
Crispy Chinese Mix	Ross	36.0	2.0	6.9	0.4	1.0
Crispy Muesli	Jordans	375	10.4	63.4	6.4	8.5
Crispy Potato Fritters,	Birds Eye					

1oz/28g	Country Club	60.0	1.0	7.5	3.0	0.3
Crispy Topped Shepherds Pie Microchef Meal	Batchelors	134	6.8	11.1	7.2	n/a
Crispy Vegetable Fingers, each	Birds Eye Country Club	45.0	1.0	5.0	2.5	0.6
Crofters' Thick Vegetable Soup	Knorr	290	11.5	54.8	2.7	n/a
Crofters' Tomato & Lentil Wholesoup, as served	Batchelors	291	13.5	53.1	2.7	13.9
Croissants		360	8.3	38.3	20.3	2.5
	International Harvest	459	8.5	36.9	30.8	1.2
Croquette Potatoes, each	Birds Eye Captain's Table	45.0	1.0	7.0	1.5	0.3
Crostinos	Findus	250	11.6	18.5	14.3	0.5
Crumble Mix	Whitworths	422	5.5	67.6	16.3	1.5
Crumpets, each	Sunblest	87.0	3.0	17.6	0.5	1.7

All amounts given per 100g/100ml unless otherwise stated

Product	*Brand*	*Calories kcal*	*Protein (g)*	*Carbo-hydrate (g)*	*Fat (g)*	*Dietary Fibre (g)*
Crunch, each	Nestlé	146	2.0	14.3	8.9	n/a
Crunch Cakes	Lyons Bakeries	510	4.5	49.0	32.9	3.8
Crunchie	Cadbury	490	5.1	67.5	18.8	n/a
Crunchy Cereal, per 40g serving with skimmed milk	Boots Shapers	180	n/a	n/a	5.2	n/a
Crunchy Cheese Wotsits, per pack	Golden Wonder	115	2.0	11.0	7.0	0.3
Crunchy Fish Bake, per pack	Birds Eye Menu Master	355	17.0	31.0	18.0	1.8
Crunchy Nut Chex	Weetabix	384	6.5	80.9	3.8	3.7
Crunchy Nut Cornflakes	Kellogg's	390	7.0	83.0	3.5	1.0
Crunchy Peanut Butter	Holland & Barrett	585	24.0	29.0	41.0	nil
	Sunpat	620	25.8	14.5	50.9	6.5
Crusha (Burgess): ***see individual flavours***						

Crusty Cobs, each	Sunblest	162	5.7	29.4	2.3	1.1
Cube Sugar, white	Tate & Lyle	400	nil	99.9	nil	nil
Cucumber, raw		10.0	0.7	1.5	0.1	0.6
Cucumber Sandwhich Spread	Heinz	183	1.2	18.5	11.5	0.4
Cullen Skink Soup	Baxters	85.0	6.6	7.9	3.2	0.5
Cultured Buttermilk	Raines	40.0	4.3	5.5	0.1	nil
Cumin, Coriander with Brinjal Pickle Partner, 28g/1oz	Kavli	118	n/a	n/a	n/a	n/a
Cup Cakes, assorted	Lyons Bakeries	357	2.3	74.8	5.2	0.4
Curacao		311	Tr	28.3	nil	nil
Curly Kale, raw		33.0	3.4	1.4	1.6	3.1
boiled		24.0	2.4	1.0	1.1	2.8
Curly Wurly	Cadbury	424	5.0	64.2	16.6	n/a

All amounts given per 100g/100ml unless otherwise stated

Product	Brand	Calories kcal	Protein (g)	Carbo-hydrate (g)	Fat (g)	Dietary Fibre (g)
Currant Buns		296	7.6	52.7	7.5	N
	Sunblest	288	8.6	50.3	5.8	2.8
Currants, dried		267	2.3	67.8	0.4	1.9
	Holland & Barrett	243	1.7	63.1	Tr	6.5
Curried Baked Beans with Sultanas	Heinz	113	5.3	19.6	1.5	4.2
Curried Beef & Vegetables	Tyne Brand	87.0	3.7	11.0	3.4	n/a
Curried Chicken Sandwich Filler	Heinz	182	5.8	7.6	14.3	0.6
Curried Chicken with Rice Soup	Heinz	55.0	1.4	6.6	2.5	0.3
Curried Fruit Chutney	Sharwood	129	1.0	30.3	0.4	2.6
Curried Mince & Vegetables	Tyne Brand	100	5.7	9.6	4.3	n/a
Curry Casserole Recipe Sauce	Knorr	91.0	1.4	13.4	3.9	n/a

Curry Concentrate	Lea & Perrins	250	Tr	33.4	12.9	n/a
Curry Cook-In-Sauce	Homepride	105	0.9	20.9	7.2	n/a
Curry Dip, 28g/1oz	Kavli	98.0	n/a	n/a	n/a	n/a
Curry Sauce	HP	137	1.6	24.0	3.8	n/a
Curry Sauce, canned		78.0	1.5	7.1	5.0	N
Curry Sauce Mix, as sold	Colman's	368	7.5	65.0	8.4	n/a
Curry Spaghetti	Crosse & Blackwell	70.0	2.0	14.4	0.5	0.6
Curry Wotsits, per pack	Golden Wonder	112	1.3	12.4	6.3	0.4
Custard						
made up with whole milk		117	3.7	16.6	4.5	Tr
made up with skimmed milk		79.0	3.8	16.8	0.1	Tr
canned		95.0	2.6	15.4	3.0	0.1
canned, low fat	Ambrosia	75.0	3.0	12.5	1.4	nil
powder	Creamola	350	0.4	92.0	0.7	n/a
ready to serve	Bird's	100	2.7	15.5	3.0	nil

All amounts given per 100g/100ml unless otherwise stated

Product	*Brand*	*Calories kcal*	*Protein (g)*	*Carbo-hydrate (g)*	*Fat (g)*	*Dietary Fibre (g)*
Custard Creams	Jacob's	483	5.3	71.7	21.2	1.3
each	Crawford's	62.0	0.8	8.2	2.9	0.2
Custard Tarts		277	6.3	32.4	14.5	1.2

D

Dairy Box Assortment	Nestlé	457	5.2	64.6	19.8	n/a
Dairy Cream Sponge	St Ivel	278	4.3	42.1	10.3	0.8
Dairy/Fat Spread (see also brands & flavours)		662	0.4	Tr	73.4	nil
Dairy Fudge, each	Trebor Bassett	42.8	0.2	6.7	1.6	nil
Dairy Ice Cream: *see Ice Cream*						
Dairylea Cheese Food Slices	Kraft	315	18.0	5.1	25.0	nil
Dairylea Cheese Spread	Kraft	280	12.2	5.8	23.0	nil
with Bacon	Kraft	280	13.0	6.0	23.0	nil
with Onion	Kraft	275	11.0	6.0	23.0	Tr
Dairylea Light Cheese Spread with Skimmed Milk	Kraft	185	15.0	6.4	11.0	nil

Product	Brand	Calories kcal	Protein (g)	Carbo-hydrate (g)	Fat (g)	Dietary Fibre (g)
Dairy Milk Chocolate	Cadbury	525	7.8	56.8	29.4	n/a
Dairy Milk Tasters	Cadbury	520	7.7	57.0	29.2	n/a
Dairy Toffee	Cravens	472	1.8	75.3	18.3	nil
Damsons						
raw (weighed with stones)		34.0	0.5	8.6	Tr	1.6
stewed with sugar		107	1.3	26.9	0.1	1.5
Dandelion & Burdock	Barr	28.0	n/a	6.7	Tr	Tr
	Idris	28.0	nil	7.5	Tr	n/a
low calorie	Barr	1.5	n/a	n/a	n/a	n/a
Danish Blue Cheese		347	20.1	Tr	29.6	nil
Danish Brown Bread	Heinz Weight Watchers	207	9.6	38.6	1.6	9.9
Danish Malted Softgrain Bread	Heinz Weight Watchers	229	10.0	44.8	1.1	3.4
Danish Pastries		374	5.8	51.3	17.6	1.6
Danish Toaster Bread	Mothers Pride	242	9.1	46.5	2.2	3.6

	Sunblest	235	7.6	45.7	2.4	2.3
Danish White Bread	Heinz Weight Watchers	225	8.6	45.4	1.0	2.7
	Sunblest	235	7.6	45.7	2.4	2.3
Dansak Classic Curry Sauce	Homepride	97.0	3.2	13.1	3.4	n/a
Dansak Curry Sauce	Uncle Ben's	108	1.9	10.8	6.2	n/a
Dark Brown Soft Sugar	Tate & Lyle	384	0.2	95.0	nil	nil
Dark Classico, each	Lyons Maid	135	1.5	13.5	8.5	n/a
Dark Treacle Cookies	Heinz Weight Watchers	420	5.3	65.9	15.1	1.8
Dates, raw, weighed with stones		227	2.8	57.1	0.2	1.5
dried		268	2.3	68.1	0.4	3.4
block	Whitworths	288	3.3	68.0	0.2	n/a
stoned	Whitworths	287	3.2	68.0	0.2	3.9
Deep Pan Pizza Bases	Napolina	1150	7.6	58.5	2.3	n/a
Delight Double Cream Alternative	Van Den Berghs	243	2.7	4.0	24.0	0.3

All amounts given per 100g/100ml unless otherwise stated

Product	*Brand*	*Calories kcal*	*Protein (g)*	*Carbo-hydrate (g)*	*Fat (g)*	*Dietary Fibre (g)*
Delight Extra Low	Van Den Berghs	223	3.6	1.6	22.5	nil
Delight Low Fat Spread	Van Den Berghs	364	2.8	0.5	39.0	nil
Delight Single Cream Alternative	Van Den Berghs	125	3.0	6.2	9.4	0.3
Delight Whipping Cream Alternative	Van Den Berghs	195	3.0	4.5	18.3	0.2
Deluxe Muesli	Holland & Barrett	356	8.9	53.2	11.1	15.4
Demerara Sugar		394	0.5	104.5	nil	nil
Derby Cheese		402	24.2	0.1	33.9	nil
Desiccated Coconut: *see Coconut*						
Dessert Top	Nestlé	291	2.4	6.0	28.8	Tr
Dessert White Sauce	Ambrosia	96.0	2.9	14.6	3.0	n/a
Dessicated Coconut	Holland & Barrett	604	5.6	6.4	62.0	23.5

Devon Custard	Ambrosia	102	2.8	15.8	3.1	n/a
low fat	Ambrosia	75.0	3.0	12.5	1.4	n/a
Dhansak Cooking Sauce	Sharwood	91.0	2.8	9.7	4.6	1.8
Diabetic Products (Boots, Dietade): ***see individual flavours***						
Diced Pineapple	Holland & Barrett	334	0.5	86.9	0.1	1.3
Dietade (Applefords): ***see individual products***						
Diet Clover	Dairy Crest	390	7.8	0.5	39.6	nil
Diet Drinks: ***see individual flavours***						
Diet Ski Yogurt (Eden Vale): ***see individual flavours***						
Digestive Biscuit	Holland & Barrett	477	5.4	66.3	21.2	nil
Digestive Biscuits						
chocolate		493	6.8	66.5	24.1	2.2
plain		471	6.3	68.6	20.9	2.2
Dijon Mustard	Colman's	156	7.7	4.3	11.0	n/a

Product	*Brand*	*Calories kcal*	*Protein (g)*	*Carbo-hydrate (g)*	*Fat (g)*	*Dietary Fibre (g)*
Dinner Supreme (Findus): ***see individual flavours***						
Dinosaur Bites	McCain	180	3.4	32.0	5.2	n/a
Dinosaurs Pasta Shapes in Tomato Sauce	Heinz	67.0	2.3	13.5	0.4	0.8
Dinosaurs with Mini Meat Boulders	Heinz	88.0	4.0	12.0	2.6	0.7
Disney Fun Pasta	Crosse & Blackwell	60.0	1.7	12.5	0.4	0.4
Disney Fun Pasta Tomato Soup	Crosse & Blackwell	70.0	1.1	10.1	2.9	0.4
Disney Pasta & Sausages	Crosse & Blackwell	95.0	3.4	10.1	4.8	0.2
Disney Pasta Bolognese	Crosse & Blackwell	70.0	3.0	10.7	1.6	0.4
Disney Pasta with Beans	Crosse & Blackwell	80.0	3.4	15.8	0.5	3.4

Disney Ravioli	Crosse & Blackwell	75.0	1.6	12.4	2.0	0.4
Ditto	Tunnock's	457	4.3	62.8	22.8	n/a
Dolmio Pasta & Pasta Sauces: ***see individual flavours***						
Dopiaza Classic Curry Sauce	Homepride	76.0	1.3	10.9	2.9	n/a
Double Choc Chip Crumble	Jacob's	493	6.6	61.3	24.7	3.4
Double Choc Club Biscuit	Jacob's	522	5.7	59.3	29.1	1.5
Double Decker	Cadbury	465	4.9	69.9	18.1	n/a
Double Gloucester Cheese		405	24.6	0.1	34.0	nil
Doublemint Chewing Gum	Wrigley	311	nil	76.0	nil	nil
Doughnuts, jam		336	5.7	48.8	14.5	N
ring		397	6.1	47.2	21.7	N
	Sunblest	375	5.1	47.9	18.1	0.8
Dream Topping, standard	Bird's	680	7.0	32.0	58.0	0.5
sugar free	Bird's	695	7.3	30.5	60.5	0.5
Dressed Crab	Young's	105	16.9	nil	14.2	nil

All amounts given per 100g/100ml unless otherwise stated

Product	*Brand*	*Calories kcal*	*Protein (g)*	*Carbo-hydrate (g)*	*Fat (g)*	*Dietary Fibre (g)*
Dried Bananas	Holland & Barrett	211	3.0	53.0	Tr	9.4
Dried Chestnuts	Holland & Barrett	344	6.7	74.6	4.1	6.8
Dried Fruit Salad	Holland & Barrett	204	3.1	51.0	Tr	15.8
	Whitworths	145	2.6	39.9	0.5	4.2
Dried Milk , skimmed, as sold		348	36.1	52.9	0.6	nil
Dried Pears	Holland & Barrett	282	3.1	67.3	2.0	6.2
Drifter	Nestlé	477	4.7	66.1	21.5	n/a
Drinking Chocolate, powder		366	5.5	77.4	6.0	N
made up with whole milk		90.0	3.4	10.6	4.1	Tr
made up with semi-skimmed milk		71.0	3.5	10.8	1.9	Tr
Dripping, beef		891	Tr	Tr	99.0	nil
Dry Ginger Ale	Schweppes	16.0	n/a	3.8	n/a	n/a

Dry Roasted Nuts, per pack	Golden Wonder	278	13.3	15.7	18.5	2.7
DSF Mustard Powder	Colman's	518	29.0	24.0	34.0	n/a
Duck						
meat only, roast		189	25.3	nil	9.7	nil
meat, fat & skin, roast		339	19.6	nil	29.0	nil
Dumplings		208	2.8	24.5	11.7	0.9
Dutch Apple Tart	McVitie's	237	3.2	34.4	9.9	0.6
Dutch Cauliflower & Broccoli Cup-A-Soup, per sachet	Batchelors	106	1.5	16.0	4.5	n/a
Dutch Cheese: ***see Edam, Gouda***						

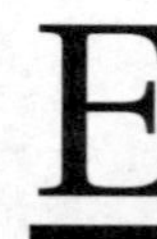

Product	*Brand*	*Calories kcal*	*Protein (g)*	*Carbo-hydrate (g)*	*Fat (g)*	*Dietary Fibre (g)*
Easter Bakewells, each	Mr Kipling	211	1.9	32.1	8.3	n/a
Easter Cakes	Mr Kipling	117	1.6	15.2	5.5	n/a
Easter Gateau	Mr Kipling	437	5.0	59.0	20.1	n/a
Easter Nests	Mr Kipling	124	1.4	15.9	6.1	n/a
Easy Cook White Rice, boiled		138	2.6	30.9	1.3	0.1
Eccles Cakes		475	3.9	59.3	26.4	1.6
Echo Margarine	Van Den Berghs	731	0.1	0.4	81.0	nil
Eclairs, frozen		396	5.6	26.1	30.6	0.8
Economy Burgers, each	Birds Eye Steakhouse	114	6.5	5.0	7.5	0.2

Economy Salad Cream	Burgess	283	1.2	7.5	27.3	nil
Edam Cheese		333	26.0	Tr	25.4	nil
Egg & Cress Four Pack Selection Sandwiches, per pack	Boots Shapers	290	n/a	n/a	n/a	n/a
Egg Fried Rice		208	4.2	25.7	10.6	0.4
Egg Mayonnaise Club Sandwiches, per pack	Boots Shapers	182	n/a	n/a	n/a	n/a
Eggplant: *see Aubergine*						
Eggs, chicken						
raw, whole		147	12.5	Tr	10.8	nil
raw, white only		36.0	9.0	Tr	Tr	nil
raw, yolk only		339	16.1	Tr	30.5	nil
boiled		147	12.5	Tr	10.8	nil
fried		179	13.6	Tr	13.9	nil
poached		147	12.5	Tr	10.8	nil
scrambled with milk		247	10.7	0.6	22.6	nil
Eggs, duck, raw, whole		163	14.3	Tr	11.8	nil

Product	*Brand*	*Calories kcal*	*Protein (g)*	*Carbo-hydrate (g)*	*Fat (g)*	*Dietary Fibre (g)*
Egg Salad Sandwiches	Boots Shapers	198	n/a	n/a	n/a	n/a
Elmlea Double Cream	Van Den Berghs	410	2.3	3.5	43.0	0.2
Elmlea Ready Whipped Cream	Van Den Berghs	256	6.3	6.3	25.0	Tr
Elmlea Single Cream	Van Den Berghs	183	3.0	4.5	17.0	0.2
Elmlea Whipping Cream	Van Den Berghs	321	3.5	3.5	33.0	0.1
English Apple Juice	Cawston Vale	42.0	0.1	10.8	Tr	n/a
English Cheddar Cheese		412	25.5	0.1	34.4	nil
English Mustard	Colman's	187	7.0	19.0	9.3	n/a
Evaporated Milk, whole		151	8.4	8.5	9.4	nil
	Carnation	160	8.2	11.5	9.0	n/a
full cream	Nestlé Ideal	160	8.2	11.5	9.0	n/a
Everton Mints	Cravens	413	0.6	89.8	5.7	nil
Extra Basil Pasta Sauce	Dolmio	58.0	0.8	7.8	2.7	n/a
Extra Chunky Vegetables						

Pasta Sauce	Dolmio	35.0	1.9	6.9	Tr	n/a
Extra Garlic Pasta Sauce	Dolmio	38.0	1.1	7.3	0.5	n/a
Extra Hot Curry Paste	Sharwood	332	4.3	12.6	29.4	5.3
Extra Strong Mints, each	Trebor Bassett	10.7	nil	2.6	nil	nil
Extra Virgin Olive Oil	Napolina	828	nil	nil	92.0	nil

All amounts given per 100g/100ml unless otherwise stated

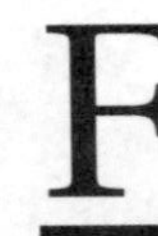

Product	Brand	Calories kcal	Protein (g)	Carbo-hydrate (g)	Fat (g)	Dietary Fibre (g)
Fab, each	Lyons Maid	99.0	0.6	16.6	3.3	n/a
Faggots		268	11.1	15.3	18.5	N
Faggots in Rich Sauce	Mr Brain's	143	7.0	13.0	7.0	n/a
Faggots in Tomato & Onion Sauce	Mr Brain's	132	6.9	10.3	5.3	n/a
Family Soft Wholemeal Bread	Allinson	222	10.8	37.0	3.4	6.5
Family Steak & Kidney Deep Pie	Ross	270	7.2	23.9	16.7	1.0
Family Wheatgerm Bread	Hovis	227	10.7	35.3	2.9	4.0
Fancy Iced Cakes		407	3.8	68.8	14.9	N

Farmhouse Baps, each	Sunblest	113	3.9	24.1	2.3	0.9
Farmhouse Beef & Vegetable Soup	Heinz	37.0	1.2	5.8	1.0	0.6
Farmhouse Chicken & Leek Soup	Knorr	415	6.5	54.6	19.0	n/a
Farmhouse Mince & Tomato Casserole Mix, as sold	Colman's	309	9.7	63.0	0.9	n/a
Farmhouse Mince & Vegetables	Tyne Brand	74.0	5.9	6.7	2.6	n/a
Farmhouse Sausage Casserole Cooking Mix	Colman's	323	7.3	n/a	0.9	n/a
Farmhouse Sausage Casserole Mix, as sold	Colman's	323	7.3	70.0	0.9	n/a
Farmhouse Vegetable Packet Soup, as served	Batchelors	239	8.4	51.4	2.6	6.1
Farmhouse Vegetable WholeSoup	Heinz	45.0	2.2	7.9	0.4	0.9

All amounts given per 100g/100ml unless otherwise stated

Product	Brand	Calories kcal	Protein (g)	Carbo-hydrate (g)	Fat (g)	Dietary Fibre (g)
Farrows Marrowfat Peas	Batchelors	82.0	5.8	18.3	0.7	n/a
Fat Free Garlic & Herb Dressing	Kraft	50.0	1.4	10.5	Tr	2.4
Fat Free Yogurt & Chive Dressing	Kraft	47.0	1.5	8.3	0.1	2.5
Fennel, Florence, raw		12.0	0.9	1.8	0.2	2.4
boiled		11.0	0.9	1.5	0.2	2.3
Feta Cheese		250	15.6	1.5	20.2	nil
Fibrewhite Bread	Mothers Pride	227	8.0	44.2	2.0	4.1
Fig Rolls	Jacob's	363	4.6	70.2	7.1	4.0
Figs, dried		209	3.3	48.6	1.5	7.5
ready to eat		122	0.4	7.2	Tr	6.9
Figs in Syrup	Libby	88.0	n/a	n/a	Tr	n/a
Filet-O-Fish, each	McDonald's	350	16.0	36.1	15.6	3.4
Fillet of Haddock with Julienne Veg.	Ross	125	13.0	3.2	6.8	0.1

Fine Blend	Nescafé	94.0	12.6	11.0	Tr	n/a
Finger Rolls, each	Sunblest	102	3.5	17.6	1.4	0.6
Finger Shortbread	McVitie's	525	6.1	63.1	27.1	2.0
Fish 'n' Chips Candy, each	Trebor Bassett	35.1	0.2	4.3	1.8	nil
Fish & Potato Bake	Ross	83.0	5.8	8.1	3.3	0.1
Fish & Tomato Gratin	Ross	120	7.3	9.3	6.2	0.4
Fish Cakes, fried		188	9.1	15.1	10.5	N
each	Birds Eye Country Club	85.0	4.5	9.0	3.5	0.2
Fish fingers fried in oil		233	13.5	17.2	12.7	0.6
grilled		214	15.1	19.3	9.0	0.7
grilled, each	Birds Eye Captain's Table	45.0	3.0	4.0	20	0.1
	Ross	186	11.5	16.3	8.6	0.7
Fish Mornay	Ross	137	6.6	11.8	7.3	0.5
Fish Paste		169	15.3	3.7	10.4	0.2

Product	*Brand*	*Calories kcal*	*Protein (g)*	*Carbo-hydrate (g)*	*Fat (g)*	*Dietary Fibre (g)*
Fish Pie		102	8.0	12.3	3.0	0.7
Fish Portions in Crispy Crumb	Ross	206	10.9	19.2	9.8	0.8
Fish Provençale with Noodles	Heinz Weight Watchers	78.0	6.2	9.4	1.7	0.7
Fish Shop Cod Fillets	Ross	76.0	17.4	nil	0.7	nil
Fish Shop Fish Fillets	Ross	257	11.8	20.1	14.6	0.6
Fish Shop Haddock Fillets	Ross	73.0	16.8	nil	0.6	nil
Fish Shop Plaice Fillets	Ross	120	10.3	21.0	0.4	0.9
Fish Steaks in Butter Sauce	Ross	93.0	9.4	2.9	4.9	0.1
Fish Steaks in Parsley Sauce	Ross	85.0	9.4	2.9	4.9	0.1
Fish Stock Cubes	Knorr	300	19.5	9.3	20.5	n/a
Fisherman's Pie with Broccoli & Sweetcorn	Findus Lean Cuisine	83.0	7.0	10.0	1.7	0.9
Fisherman's Pottage	Baxters	41.0	3.7	3.3	1.6	0.1
Five Fruit 'C'	Libby	40.0	0.1	10.0	Tr	Tr

Five Fruits Fruit Burst	Del Monte	46.0	0.2	11.1	Tr	n/a
Flageolet Beans	Batchelors	98.0	7.1	21.5	0.8	n/a
Flake	Cadbury	530	8.1	55.7	30.7	n/a
Flake Cakes, each	Cadbury	141	2.0	17.4	6.6	n/a
Flaky Pastry: ***see Pastry***						
Flapjacks		484	4.5	60.4	26.6	2.7
Flapjack Slice	Peek Frean	319	5.5	61.3	26.1	2.9
Flintstones in Tomato Sauce	Heinz	58.0	1.9	11.7	0.4	0.6
Flora, baking	Van Den Berghs	736	Tr	Tr	82.0	n/a
Flora Cream Alternative						
double	Van Den Berghs	69.0	0.4	0.5	7.3	n/a
single	Van Den Berghs	30.0	0.5	0.7	2.8	n/a
Flora Sunflower Oil	Van Den Berghs	900	nil	nil	100	nil
Flora Sunflower Spread	Van Den Berghs	635	0.2	1.0	70.0	nil
extra light	Van Den Berghs	368	3.7	0.5	39.0	nil
reduced salt	Van Den Berghs	635	0.2	1.0	70.0	nil

Product	*Brand*	*Calories kcal*	*Protein (g)*	*Carbo-hydrate (g)*	*Fat (g)*	*Dietary Fibre (g)*
Florida Sponge	Mr Kipling	357	4.4	64.4	9.1	n/a
Florida Spring Vegetable Soup	Knorr	283	8.9	47.0	6.6	n/a
Florida Wafer	Tunnock's	519	5.1	64.0	29.0	n/a
Flour, wheat						
brown		323	12.6	68.5	1.8	6.4
white, breadmaking		341	11.5	75.3	1.4	3.1
white, plain		341	9.4	77.7	1.3	3.1
white, self-raising		330	8.9	75.6	1.2	3.1
wholemeal		310	12.7	63.9	2.2	9.0
Forest Fruit Juice Drink	Ribena	52.0	Tr	13.9	n/a	n/a
Forest Fruits Yogurt	St Ivel Shape	41.0	4.6	5.5	0.0	0.1
Four Cheese Pasta Choice	Crosse & Blackwell	400	14.3	61.6	10.6	2.6
Fox's Glacier Fruits	Nestlé	381	nil	95.3	nil	n/a
Fox's Glacier Mints	Nestlé	386	nil	96.4	nil	n/a

Frankfurters		274	9.5	3.0	25.0	0.1
Frappe, ready to drink	Nescafé	64.0	2.7	7.3	2.7	nil
Fred Bear Beans & Pasta Shapes	Crosse & Blackwell	81.0	3.4	15.8	0.5	3.4
Freedent Mint Chewing Gum	Wrigley	311	nil	75.0	nil	nil
French Bean & Almond Soup	Baxters	63.0	1.6	3.5	4.9	1.3
French Beans: *see Green Beans/French Beans*						
French Bread Pizza: *see individual flavours*						
French Chasseur Sauce	Campbell's	48.0	0.9	8.6	1.2	n/a
French Chicken & Asparagus Cup-A-Soup, per sachet	Batchelors	100	1.0	15.6	4.2	n/a
French Classic Yellow Mustard	Colman's	73.0	4.3	2.6	4.2	n/a
French Dressing		649	0.3	0.1	72.1	nil
French Fancies, each	Mr Kipling	107	0.6	19.8	2.8	n/a
French Fries, regular, per portion	McDonald's	267	3.2	31.2	14.3	5.8

Product	*Brand*	*Calories kcal*	*Protein (g)*	*Carbo-hydrate (g)*	*Fat (g)*	*Dietary Fibre (g)*
French Mix Vegetables	Ross	21.0	1.7	5.1	0.1	1.8
French Mushroom & Herb Slim-A-Soup Special, per sachet	Batchelors	60.0	0.8	9.7	2.5	n/a
French Mustard	Burgess	144	6.8	12.6	6.0	0.2
	Colman's	104	6.3	n/a	7.0	n/a
French Mustard & Garlic Soup of the World	Knorr	431	8.2	51.9	21.2	n/a
French Onion Soup	Batchelors	47.0	1.1	3.8	3.0	n/a
	Baxters	24.0	0.9	5.4	Tr	Tr
	Knorr	311	7.6	60.0	4.5	n/a
French Potato & Leek Cup-A-Soup, per sachet	Batchelors	109	1.4	16.7	4.5	n/a
French Provençale Sauce	Campbell's	50.0	1.0	7.8	1.6	n/a
French Sandwich Cake	Lyons Bakeries	368	3.5	56.4	13.9	1.0
French Soupe Paysanne						

Soup of the World	Knorr	292	10.4	51.1	5.1	n/a
French Vinaigrette Dressing	Kraft	425	0.8	4.2	44.5	0.1
French White Wine & Dill Cooking Sauce	Heinz Weight Watchers	41.0	1.1	8.5	0.1	0.4
Fresh Garden Mint Sauce	Colman's	30.0	1.4	2.6	0.1	n/a
Freshwater King Prawns	Lyons Seafoods	70.0	16.8	nil	0.3	n/a
Fried Bread: *see Bread, fried*						
Friij Chocolate Milkshake	Dairy Crest	79.0	4.2	11.5	1.8	nil
Fromage frais						
fruit		131	6.8	13.8	5.8	Tr
plain		113	6.8	5.7	7.1	nil
very low fat		58.0	7.7	6.8	0.2	Tr
Frosted Chex	Weetabix	375	6.1	83.7	1.7	3.5
Frosties	Kellogg's	380	5.0	88.0	0.5	0.6
Fruit 'n' Fibre	Kellogg's	350	9.0	67.0	6.0	7.0
Fruit & Nut Bournville	Cadbury	495	5.7	57.6	23.0	n/a

Product	Brand	Calories kcal	Protein (g)	Carbo-hydrate (g)	Fat (g)	Dietary Fibre (g)
Fruit & Nut Bran	Weetabix	319	12.6	49.3	8.0	18.3
Fruit & Nut Chocolate	Cadbury	475	7.8	56.0	24.5	n/a
Fruit & Nut Harvest Chewy Bar, each	Quaker	103	2.1	14.4	3.8	0.8
Fruit & Nut Tasters	Cadbury	505	9.3	52.1	29.0	n/a
Fruit Burst Drinks (Del Monte): *see individual flavours*						
Fruit Cake						
plain, retail		354	5.1	57.9	12.9	N
rich, recipe		341	3.8	59.6	11.0	1.7
rich, iced		356	4.1	62.7	11.4	1.7
wholemeal		363	6.0	52.8	15.7	2.4
Fruit Club Biscuits	Jacob's	496	5.7	62.1	25.0	1.8
Fruit Cocktail						
canned in juice		57.0	0.4	14.8	Tr	1.0
	Libby	52.0	0.2	12.7	Tr	0.3
canned in syrup		77.0	0.4	20.1	Tr	1.0
	Libby	74.0	0.2	18.2	Tr	0.4

Fruit Cocktail Luxury Trifle	St Ivel	182	2.6	23.5	2.6	0.6
Fruit Drops	Cravens	386	2.0	70.3	22.7	0.5
Fruited Teacakes, each	Sunblest	151	5.4	25.6	3.0	1.6
Fruitetts	G. Payne & Co	415	6.1	91.0	3.0	n/a
Fruit Flapjack	Holland & Barrett	468	4.8	50.8	24.1	4.8
Fruit Fromage Frais, creamy	Chambourcy	122	5.8	16.2	4.2	n/a
Fruit Fromage Frais, very low fat	Chambourcy	83.0	6.8	13.9	0.4	n/a
Fruit Gums		172	1.0	44.8	nil	nil
	Nestlé	344	0.5	85.5	nil	n/a
Fruitini Mixed Fruit in Creamy Tropical Sauce	Del Monte	70.0	1.2	14.0	1.1	n/a
Fruitini Peaches in Light Syrup	Del Monte	58.0	0.4	15.0	0.1	n/a
Fruitini Pineapple in Light Syrup	Del Monte	58.0	0.4	15.0	0.1	n/a

Product	*Brand*	*Calories kcal*	*Protein (g)*	*Carbo-hydrate (g)*	*Fat (g)*	*Dietary Fibre (g)*
Fruit Jaspers	McVitie's	499	5.4	65.6	23.6	3.4
Fruit Mousse		137	4.5	18.0	5.7	N
Fruit Pastil Lolly, each	Nestlé	66.0	Tr	14.9	nil	n/a
Fruit Pastilles	Nestlé/Rowntree	350	4.3	83.2	nil	n/a
Fruit Pie, one crust		186	2.0	28.7	7.9	1.7
pastry top & bottom		260	3.0	34.0	13.3	1.8
individual		369	4.3	56.7	15.5	N
wholemeal, one crust		183	2.6	26.6	8.1	2.7
Fruit Pie Selection, each	Mr Kipling	241	2.1	39.2	8.4	n/a
Fruit Pies (Lyons): ***see individual flavours***						
Fruit Salad Chews, each	Trebor Bassett	15.4	nil	3.3	0.2	nil
Fruit Salad, homemade, dried		19.0	1.1	3.0	0.4	1.5
Fruit Sauce	Lea & Perrins	151	1.5	36.2	Tr	n/a
Fruit Scones, each	Sunblest	161	3.2	26.9	4.5	0.9

Fruit Shortcake	McVitie's	488	5.1	70.6	19.5	2.6
Fruit Shortcake Biscuit	Holland & Barrett	490	4.6	64.8	23.6	nil
Fruits o' Forest Bio Splitpot, per pack	Boots Shapers	79.0	n/a	n/a	0.2	n/a
Fruits of the Forest Cheesecake	McVitie's	302	4.5	31.9	17.7	0.6
Fruits of the Forest in Syrup	Libby	82.0	0.4	20.2	Tr	0.5
Fruits of the Forest Jam, reduced sugar	Heinz Weight Watchers	127	0.3	31.2	0.1	0.7
Fruits of the Forest Pavlova	McVitie's	293	2.7	43.6	12.0	Tr
Fruit Sponge Pudding Mix, made up, per serving	Homepride	342	4.5	75.5	14.5	n/a
Fruit Sundaes Selection, each	Mr Kipling	184	1.1	28.8	7.2	n/a
Fruity Barbecue Sauce	HP	136	0.9	31.0	0.9	n/a

All amounts given per 100g/100ml unless otherwise stated

Product	*Brand*	*Calories kcal*	*Protein (g)*	*Carbo-hydrate (g)*	*Fat (g)*	*Dietary Fibre (g)*
Fruity Sauce	Colman's	95.0	0.9	n/a	0.2	n/a
	HP	117	1.1	27.0	0.6	n/a
Fudge	Cadbury	445	3.6	71.9	16.2	n/a
Fudge Harvest Chewy Bar, each	Quaker	102	1.5	16.1	3.0	0.6
Fudge Slice	California Cake & Cookie Ltd	438	5.5	69.0	22.0	n/a

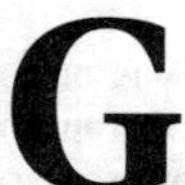

Galaxy Caramel	Mars	488	5.3	60.1	25.1	n/a
Galaxy Double Nut/Raisin	Mars	534	8.4	55.7	30.8	n/a
Galaxy Hazlenut	Mars	572	7.7	48.5	38.6	n/a
Galaxy Milk Chocolate Bar	Mars	488	5.3	60.1	25.1	n/a
Galaxy Minstrels	Mars	491	6.0	69.5	21.0	n/a
Galaxy Ripple	Mars	532	9.0	56.6	30.0	n/a
Gammon: *see Bacon, gammon*						
Garden Peas	Ross	72.0	6.0	14.5	0.8	4.3
Garden Peas in Water						
no sugar	Batchelors	64.0	4.2	10.5	0.4	3.9
with sugar	Batchelors	64.0	4.1	12.0	0.4	n/a

Product	*Brand*	*Calories kcal*	*Protein (g)*	*Carbo-hydrate (g)*	*Fat (g)*	*Dietary Fibre (g)*
Garden Pea with Mint Soup	Baxters	32.0	1.6	6.3	0.3	1.8
Garden Vegetable Soup	Crosse & Blackwell	39.0	1.0	7.2	0.7	0.9
Garlic, raw		98.0	7.9	16.3	0.6	4.1
Garlic & Herb Dip, per pack	Boots Shapers	159	n/a	n/a	13.0	n/a
Garlic & Herb Sandwich	Jacob's	488	8.4	59.5	24.0	1.7
Garlic & Herb Sauce Mix, as sold	Colman's	413	13.0	47.0	19.0	n/a
Garlic & Herbs Stuffing Mix	Knorr	426	11.2	64.5	13.7	n/a
Garlic & Mint Dip, 28g/1oz	Kavli	98.0	n/a	n/a	n/a	n/a
Garlic & Spring Onion Sauce	Lea & Perrins	74.0	1.4	16.1	0.5	n/a
Garlic Crackerbread	Ryvita	373	10.9	75.8	2.9	4.6
Garlic Dip, 28g/1oz	Kavli	98.0	n/a	n/a	n/a	n/a
Garlic Mayonnaise	Hellmanns	720	1.1	1.3	79.1	n/a

Garlic Mushroom Soup, per pack	Boots Shapers	36.00	n/a	n/a	1.2	n/a
Garlic Partner, 28g/1oz	Kavli	117	n/a	n/a	n/a	n/a
Garlic Pâté, per pack	Boots Shapers	131	n/a	n/a	8.3	n/a
Garlic Prawnnaise	Lyons Seafoods	410	6.1	1.9	41.8	n/a
Garlic Puree	Sharwood	63.0	3.4	13.3	0.3	2.4
Garlic Sauce	Lea & Perrins	323	2.0	10.4	30.4	1.5
Gateau		337	5.7	43.4	16.8	0.4
German Mustard	Colman's	98.0	5.3	n/a	7.5	n/a
Ghee						
butter		898	Tr	Tr	99.8	nil
palm		897	Tr	Tr	99.7	nil
vegetable		898	Tr	Tr	99.8	nil
Gherkins, pickled		14.0	0.9	2.6	0.1	1.2
raw		12.0	1.0	1.8	0.1	0.8
Giant Cornish Pastie	Ross	228	6.5	24.5	12.0	1.0

All amounts given per 100g/100ml unless otherwise stated

Product	Brand	Calories kcal	Protein (g)	Carbo-hydrate (g)	Fat (g)	Dietary Fibre (g)
Giant Minced Beef & Onion Pastie	Ross	259	6.0	28.0	14.2	1.2
Giant Minestrone Soup	Heinz Big Soup	48.0	1.9	7.8	1.0	1.0
Giant Size Sausage Rolls	Kraft	320	6.6	24.7	22.3	n/a
Giardinera Ragu Pizza Topping	Batchelors	58.0	1.7	7.8	2.3	1.6
Gin: *see Spirits*						
Ginger & Orange Sauce	Lea & Perrins	69.0	0.3	14.6	1.0	n/a
Ginger Beer	Idris	49.0	nil	12.2	nil	n/a
	Schweppes	34.7	n/a	8.4	n/a	n/a
Gingernut Biscuits		456	5.6	79.1	15.2	1.4
	McVitie's	460	5.2	75.4	15.1	1.7
Ginger Root, raw		38.0	1.4	7.2	0.6	N
Ginger Sauce	Lea & Perrins	110	0.2	26.0	0.5	n/a
Ginger Slices, each	Mr Kipling	95.0	1.2	18.8	1.7	n/a

Ginger Wafer	Holland & Barrett	490	4.7	64.8	23.6	nil
Gipsy Creams	McVitie's	514	4.9	62.8	26.9	2.6
Glacé Cherries: *see Cherries*						
Glacé Ginger	Whitworths	303	0.1	74.2	0.7	Tr
Glazed Chicken	Findus Lean Cuisine	105	10.0	9.6	3.0	1.3
Glazed Fruit Tartlets, each	Mr Kipling	201	1.8	31.6	7.0	n/a
Glazed Mince Tartlets, each	Mr Kipling	218	2.2	31.2	8.2	n/a
Glazed Chicken Platter, per meal	Birds Eye Healthy Options	345	32.0	32.0	9.5	4.0
Globe Artichoke: *see Artichoke, globe*						
Goats Milk		60.0	3.1	4.4	3.5	nil
Goats Milk Yogurt	Holland & Barrett	65.0	3.8	2.9	4.8	n/a

Product	*Brand*	*Calories kcal*	*Protein (g)*	*Carbo-hydrate (g)*	*Fat (g)*	*Dietary Fibre (g)*
Gold Blend	Nescafé	89.0	10.3	11.0	Tr	n/a
Gold Cappuccino, each	Nestlé	272	17.8	24.2	3.7	n/a
Golden Calamari	Young's	299	13.7	15.8	20.4	0.7
Golden Crackles	Kellogg's	390	7.0	81.0	4.0	1.5
Golden Crisp	Cadbury	485	6.4	64.5	22.2	n/a
Golden Crisps	Kellogg's	370	9.0	70.0	7.0	4.0
Golden Crown, light	Kraft	546	0.2	1.2	60.0	nil
Golden Crown, spreadable	Kraft	653	0.3	1.0	72.0	nil
Golden Crumble	Jacob's	466	5.5	65.1	20.3	3.0
Golden Cup	Nestlé	476	5.0	61.6	23.3	n/a
Golden Garlic Prawns	Young's	223	10.0	19.6	12.0	0.8
Golden Hake Fillets	Ross	256	9.0	17.4	17.0	0.7
Golden King Prawns	Young's	241	8.7	15.6	16.3	0.7
Golden Lemon Sole Goujons	Young's	246	10.9	26.4	11.2	1.1

Golden Oat Club Biscuit	Jacob's	505	6.5	60.0	26.5	2.2
Golden Pea Soup	Baxters	58.0	2.8	8.6	1.7	1.4
Golden Prawn Nuggets	Young's	175	11.5	11.1	9.6	0.5
Golden Savoury Rice	Batchelors	434	12.5	95.2	4.0	1.4
Golden Scampi in Breadcrumbs	Young's	172	9.4	22.1	5.5	0.9
Golden Sweetcorn	Del Monte	101	3.0	22.2	0.6	n/a
Golden Syrup		298	0.3	79.0	nil	nil
Golden Syrup Microbake Mix	Homepride	330	3.5	63.5	7.0	n/a
Golden Vegetable Cup-A-Soup, per sachet	Batchelors	75.0	1.1	13.6	2.2	n/a
Golden Vegetable Low Calorie Soup	Knorr	296	9.2	60.5	1.9	n/a
Golden Vegetable Quick Soup	Knorr	450	6.6	45.0	27.1	n/a
Golden Vegetable Slim-A-Soup, per sachet	Batchelors	38.0	0.8	8.9	0.2	n/a

All amounts given per 100g/100ml unless otherwise stated

Product	Brand	Calories kcal	Protein (g)	Carbo-hydrate (g)	Fat (g)	Dietary Fibre (g)
Golden Vegetable Soup	Knorr	344	10.4	58.5	7.6	n/a
per pack	Boots Shapers	40.00	n/a	n/a	1.1	n/a
Golden Whitebait	Young's	338	13.3	17.1	24.4	0.7
Gold Margarine	St Ivel	383	5.5	2.6	39.0	nil
lowest fat	St Ivel	264	6.0	3.7	25.0	nil
unsalted	St Ivel	387	6.0	3.0	39.0	nil
Gold Margarine Sunflower	St Ivel	367	6.0	3.1	36.8	nil
Goose, roast, meat only		319	29.3	nil	22.4	nil
Gooseberries						
raw		54.0	0.7	12.9	0.3	2.4
stewed with sugar		73.0	0.4	18.5	0.2	2.0
green, stewed without sugar		16.0	0.9	2.5	0.3	1.9
Gouda Cheese		375	24.0	Tr	31.0	nil
Goulash Cook-In-Sauce	Homepride	58.0	1.1	7.5	2.6	n/a
Gourmet King Prawns	Lyons Seafoods	51.0	12.0	nil	0.5	n/a

Granary Bread: *see Bread*						
Granary Malted Brown Bread	Hovis	230	9.6	43.1	2.1	4.8
Grannies Cake	Lyons Bakeries	421	4.5	52.0	21.6	1.2
Granulated Sugar	Tate & Lyle	400	nil	99.9	nil	nil
Grapefruit, raw, flesh only		30.0	0.8	6.8	0.1	1.3
canned in juice		30.0	0.6	7.3	Tr	0.4
canned in syrup		60.0	0.5	15.5	Tr	0.6
Grapefruit & Orange in Syrup	Libby	77.0	0.5	18.8	Tr	0.3
Grapefruit & Pineapple Drink	Tango	44.0	n/a	11.8	n/a	n/a
no added sugar, diluted	Robinsons	12.0	0.1	1.7	Tr	n/a
Grapefruit 'C'	Libby	36.0	0.2	8.8	Tr	0.3
Grapefruit Juice, unsweetened		33.0	0.4	8.3	0.1	Tr
	Britvic 55	50.0	0.5	13.3	n/a	n/a
	Del Monte	35.0	0.5	8.8	Tr	n/a

All amounts given per 100g/100ml unless otherwise stated

Product	*Brand*	*Calories kcal*	*Protein (g)*	*Carbo-hydrate (g)*	*Fat (g)*	*Dietary Fibre (g)*
Grapefruit Segments in Syrup	Libby	78.0	0.5	18.9	Tr	0.3
Grapefruit with Apple Juice	Cawston Vale	42.0	0.2	10.6	Tr	n/a
Grape Juice, unsweetened		46.0	0.3	11.7	0.1	nil
red, sparkling	Schloer	49.0	Tr	13.1	n/a	n/a
white	Schloer	48.0	Tr	12.9	n/a	n/a
white, sparkling	Schloer	49.0	Tr	13.1	n/a	n/a
Grape Nuts	Bird's	346	10.5	79.9	0.5	n/a
Grapes, black/white, seedless		60.0	0.4	15.4	0.1	0.7
Gravy Browning	Burgess	72.0	3.3	14.7	nil	nil
	Crosse & Blackwell	192	Tr	48.0	nil	nil
Gravy Instant Granules		462	4.4	40.6	32.5	Tr
made up with water		33.0	0.3	2.9	2.4	Tr
Greek Pastries (sweet)		322	4.7	40.0	17.0	N

Greek Style Raspberry Yogurt, per pack	Boots Shapers	126	n/a	n/a	4.5	n/a
Greek Style Salad Sandwiches, per pack	Boots Shapers	178	n/a	n/a	n/a	n/a
Greek Style Strawberry Yogurt, per pack	Boots Shapers	130	n/a	n/a	4.5	n/a
Greek Style Vanilla Yogurt, per pack	Boots Shapers	126	n/a	n/a	4.5	n/a
Greek Yogurt: *see Yogurt*						
Green & Red Pepper Ragu Sauce	Batchelors	79.0	1.9	11.9	2.9	n/a
Green & Red Peppers Ragu	Brooke Bond	79.0	1.9	11.9	2.9	n/a
Green Beans/French Beans						
raw		24.0	1.9	3.2	0.5	2.2
boiled		22.0	1.8	2.9	0.5	2.4
frozen, boiled		25.0	1.7	4.7	0.1	4.1
canned		22.0	1.5	4.1	0.1	2.6
Green Butterfly	Fussell's	160	8.2	11.5	9.0	n/a

Product	*Brand*	*Calories kcal*	*Protein (g)*	*Carbo-hydrate (g)*	*Fat (g)*	*Dietary Fibre (g)*
Green Chilli & Garlic Poppadums	Sharwood	274	19.9	43.3	1.6	9.7
Greengages						
raw (weighed with stones)		34.0	0.5	8.6	Tr	1.6
stewed with sugar		107	1.3	26.9	0.1	1.5
Green Label Chutney Sauce	Sharwood	222	1.0	44.8	0.3	1.4
Green Lentils: *see Lentils*						
Green Peppers: *see Peppers*						
Greens, spring: *see Spring Greens*						
Grilled Chicken Golden Lights, per pack	Golden Wonder	97.0	1.1	13.7	4.2	0.7
Grillsteaks, grilled		305	22.1	0.5	23.9	Tr
	Ross	315	15.9	nil	28.0	nil
value, each	Birds Eye Steakhouse	185	11.0	8.5	12.0	0.3
Groundnuts: *see Peanuts*						

Ground Rice	Whitworths	361	6.5	86.8	1.0	0.5
Grouse, roast		173	31.3	nil	5.3	nil
Guava, Melon & Passionfruit Jam	Baxters	210	Tr	53.0	Tr	1.4
Guavas						
raw		26.0	0.8	5.0	0.5	3.7
canned in syrup		60.0	0.4	15.7	Tr	n/a
Gumbo: ***see Okra***						

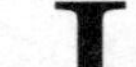

Product	*Brand*	*Calories kcal*	*Protein (g)*	*Carbo-hydrate (g)*	*Fat (g)*	*Dietary Fibre (g)*
Haddock						
steamed, flesh only		98.0	22.8	nil	0.8	nil
in crumbs, fried in oil		174	21.4	3.6	8.3	0.2
smoked, steamed, flesh only		101	23.3	nil	0.9	nil
Haddock & Prawn Crumble	Ross	181	8.7	12.6	11.2	0.5
Haddock Bake	Ross	142	7.7	11.9	7.3	0.5
Haddock Fillet Fish Fingers	Findus	205	12.0	16.5	10.0	0.2
each	Birds Eye Captain's Table	50.0	4.0	5.0	2.0	0.2
Haddock Light Crispy Fillet Steaks	Findus	215	12.4	16.7	11.2	0.6
Haddock Steaks in Butter Sauce	Ross	90.0	10.2	2.9	4.2	0.1

Haddock Steaks in Crispy Crunch Crumb, each	Birds Eye Captain's Table	225	14.0	13.0	14.0	0.9
Haddock Steaks in Natural Crumb	Ross	189	11.2	13.4	10.3	0.6
Haggis, boiled		310	10.7	19.2	21.7	N
Halibut, steamed, flesh only		131	23.8	nil	4.0	nil
Ham, canned		120	18.4	nil	5.1	nil
Ham & Beef Pâté	Shippams	189	15.1	1.7	13.5	n/a
Ham & Butterbean Soup	Heinz Wholesoup	52.0	2.2	6.7	1.9	1.3
Ham & Cheese Soup	Campbell's	60.0	1.3	3.7	4.5	n/a
Ham & Cheese Toast Topper	Heinz	104	8.3	7.1	4.8	nil
Ham & Mushroom French Bread Pizza	Heinz Weight Watchers	145	11.7	15.0	4.3	2.5
Ham & Mushroom Pizza	San Marco	227	11.4	29.5	7.5	1.1
5 inch	McCain	194	9.2	23.3	5.7	n/a
Ham & Mushroom Pizza Rolla	McCain	196	9.4	24.0	7.6	n/a

All amounts given per 100g/100ml unless otherwise stated

Product	*Brand*	*Calories kcal*	*Protein (g)*	*Carbo-hydrate (g)*	*Fat (g)*	*Dietary Fibre (g)*
Ham & Mushroom Tagliatelle Microchef Meal	Batchelors	119	5.1	10.2	6.4	n/a
Ham & Pineapple French Bread Pizza	Heinz Weight Watchers	148	11.5	15.9	4.3	2.5
Ham & Pineapple Single Serve Pizza	McCain	205	11.9	29.0	5.4	n/a
Ham & Pork, chopped, canned		275	14.4	1.4	23.6	0.3
Hamburger, each	McDonald's	244	13.9	27.7	8.6	2.7
Hamburger Buns		264	9.1	48.8	5.0	1.5
Ham Pâté	Shippams	179	17.4	3.3	10.8	n/a
Ham Salad Bap, each	Boots Shapers	184	n/a	n/a	n/a	n/a
Ham Sandwich Filler	Heinz	187	5.2	9.4	14.3	0.3
Ham Stock Cubes	Knorr	260	7.9	20.4	16.3	n/a
Handy Wheatgerm Bread	Hovis	235	11.1	40.7	3.1	4.7
Hard Cheese, average		405	24.7	0.1	34.0	nil

Hard Cheese, reduced fat	Heinz Weight Watchers	297	27.0	nil	21.0	nil
Haricot Beans, dried, boiled		95.0	6.6	17.2	0.5	6.1
Harvest Chicken & Lentil Wholesoup, as served	Batchelors	376	12.0	50.3	14.2	9.8
Harvest Crispy Clusters	Quaker	474	8.7	65.3	20.5	3.6
Harvest Crunch	Quaker	450	8.1	65.6	16.9	4.5
Harvest Thick Vegetable Soup	Crosse & Blackwell	43.0	1.6	7.9	0.6	1.1
Hash Browns	McCain	190	3.0	24.0	9.8	n/a
	McDonald's	135	1.2	15.1	7.8	2.1
Hawaiian American Sauce	Heinz	103	0.9	24.6	0.2	0.6
Hawaiian Crunch	Mornflake	401	11.0	60.0	13.0	6.5
Hazlenut Chocolate Multipack, per pack	Boots Shapers	218	n/a	n/a	5.1	n/a
Hazelnut Chocolate Squares	Mornflake	443	5.3	65.6	15.2	3.6
Hazlenut Munchies	Nestlé	500	6.4	56.3	27.7	n/a

All amounts given per 100g/100ml unless otherwise stated

Product	*Brand*	*Calories kcal*	*Protein (g)*	*Carbo-hydrate (g)*	*Fat (g)*	*Dietary Fibre (g)*
Hazelnuts, kernel only		650	14.1	6.0	63.5	6.5
Hazlenut with Herbs Stuffing Mix	Knorr	443	11.3	61.0	17.1	n/a
Healthy Balance Baked Beans	Crosse & Blackwell	90.0	5.0	16.1	0.4	5.2
Healthy Balance Ketchup	Crosse & Blackwell	93.0	1.8	20.2	0.3	0.4
Healthy Balance Tomato Ketchup	Crosse & Blackwell	93.0	1.8	20.2	0.3	0.4
Healthy Choice Baked Beans	HP	65.0	4.5	10.6	0.5	3.7
Heart						
ox, stewed		179	31.4	nil	5.9	nil
sheep, roast		237	26.1	nil	14.7	nil
Hearty Beef & Veg. Packet Soup, as served	Batchelors	233	8.7	46.6	3.7	5.3
Herb & Garlic Pâté	Tartex	230	7.5	10.0	18.0	n/a

Herb & Garlic Pitta Bread	International Harvest	248	8.5	49.2	1.9	2.8
Herb Pâté	Tartex	230	7.0	10.0	18.5	n/a
per tub	Vessen	109	3.1	5.4	8.0	0.1
Herring						
raw		234	16.8	nil	18.5	nil
fried, flesh only		234	23.1	1.5	15.1	N
grilled, flesh only		199	20.4	nil	13.0	nil
Hibran Bread	Vitbe	219	12.6	35.0	3.2	6.8
Hickory Nuts: *see Pecan Nuts*						
Hi-Fibre Biscuits	Itona	316	9.4	43.2	11.7	10.0
Hi-Fibre Biscuits with Date Syrup	Itona	387	10.3	48.2	18.5	12.3
High Bake Water Biscuits	Jacob's	408	10.3	75.0	7.4	3.1
High Fibre Corn Flakes	Ryvita	349	10.6	72.8	1.7	9.2
High Fibre Muesli	Holland & Barrett	346	10.1	60.8	7.4	n/a

Product	*Brand*	*Calories kcal*	*Protein (g)*	*Carbo-hydrate (g)*	*Fat (g)*	*Dietary Fibre (g)*
High Juice Orange, per pack	Boots Shapers	42.0	n/a	n/a	Tr	n/a
Highlander's Broth	Baxters	45.0	1.6	6.7	1.5	0.7
Highland Lentil Soup	Knorr	329	17.1	51.6	6.0	n/a
Highland Lentil Wholesoup, as served	Batchelors	332	16.7	59.3	3.1	14.3
HiGrain Bread	Vitbe	235	9.2	2.0	3.3	3.5
Hi-Juice 66	Schweppes	52.0	n/a	12.2	n/a	n/a
HiLite Bran Bread	Vitbe	222	10.2	39.1	2.8	5.5
Hilo Crackers	Rakusen	349	11.0	74.0	1.0	8.0
Hippotots Fromage Frais Dessert, all flavours	Chambourcy	192	5.6	24.3	8.0	Tr
Hob Nob Bars	McVitie's	523	6.4	61.6	27.9	2.8
Hoi Sin Chinese Spare Rib Sauce	Sharwood	182	2.8	38.3	2.4	1.9
Hollandaise Sauce Dry Mix, as sold	Crosse & Blackwell	392	10.0	50.3	6.8	1.6

Honey, comb		281	0.6	74.4	4.6	nil
in jars		288	0.4	76.4	nil	nil
	Holland & Barrett	300	0.4	78.0	n/a	n/a
Honey & Almond Crunchy Bar	Jordans	465	8.8	56.1	22.8	6.0
Honey & Mustard Chicken Tonight Sauce	Batchelors	119	1.0	16.0	5.7	n/a
Honey & Mustard Dressing	Kraft	450	10.5	9.5	44.5	0.1
Honey & Nut Cornflakes	Sunblest	397	7.5	83.3	3.8	2.1
Honey Chicken Casserole Mix, as sold	Colman's	321	3.1	75.0	0.7	n/a
Honeycomb: *see Honey, comb*						
Honey Crunchy Cereal	Holland & Barrett	361	10.5	60.0	12.0	14.0
Honeydew Melon: *see Melon*						
Honey Nut Loops	Kellogg's	380	8.0	76.0	4.5	5.0

Product	*Brand*	*Calories kcal*	*Protein (g)*	*Carbo-hydrate (g)*	*Fat (g)*	*Dietary Fibre (g)*
Honey Oatbran Bar	Jordan's	151	3.4	18.9	6.9	2.3
Honey Roast Ham Triple Pack Sandwiches, per pack	Boots Shapers	296	n/a	n/a	n/a	n/a
Hongroise Pour Over Sauce	Baxters	108	3.2	9.0	6.7	0.2
Horlicks Chocolate Malted Food Drink	SmithKline Beecham	404	11.0	74.1	7.0	5.1
Horlicks Hot Chocolate Drink	SmithKline Beecham	401	16.1	65.5	8.3	3.8
Horlicks Low Fat Instant Powder		373	17.4	72.9	3.3	N
made up with water		51.0	2.4	10.1	0.5	Tr
Horlicks Powder		378	12.4	78.0	4.0	N
made up with whole milk		99.0	4.2	12.7	3.9	Tr
made up with semi-skimmed milk		81.0	4.3	12.9	1.9	Tr
Horseradish Mustard	Colman's	185	6.5	22.0	7.2	n/a
Horseradish Relish	Colman's	105	1.8	9.3	5.5	n/a

Horseradish Sauce		153	2.5	17.9	8.4	2.5
Hot 'n' Spicy Prawns	Lyons Seafoods	275	6.5	32.1	14.3	n/a
Hot Beef Madras Pots of the World	Golden Wonder	404	11.5	59.1	13.5	n/a
Hot Chilli Chinese Pouring Sauce	Sharwood	120	0.5	29.4	0.6	1.3
Hot Chilli Sauce	Heinz	102	2.0	23.4	0.1	1.2
Hot Cross Buns		310	7.4	58.5	6.8	1.7
Hot Curry Paste	Sharwood	346	5.5	12.6	30.4	6.8
Hot Horseradish Sauce	Burgess	129	2.4	12.1	6.9	2.0
Hot Pepper & Lime Sauce	Lea & Perrins	47.0	0.2	10.7	0.3	n/a
Hot Pepper Sauce	Lea & Perrins	112	1.0	24.5	1.2	n/a
Hot Pot		114	9.4	10.1	4.5	1.2
Hot Tomato Ketchup	Heinz	101	1.3	23.8	0.1	0.8
Houmous: ***see Hummus***						

All amounts given per 100g/100ml unless otherwise stated

Product	*Brand*	*Calories kcal*	*Protein (g)*	*Carbo-hydrate (g)*	*Fat (g)*	*Dietary Fibre (g)*
Hovis Bread: ***see types of bread***						
Hovis Cracker	Jacob's	455	9.5	62.3	18.6	2.6
HP Sauce	HP	100	1.1	27.0	0.5	n/a
Hubba Bubba Bubble Gum, all flavours	Wrigley	300	nil	74.0	nil	nil
Hula Hoops: ***see Potato Hoops***						
Hummus		187	7.6	11.6	12.6	2.4
Hycal Juice, ready to drink, all flavours	SmithKline Beecham	243	nil	64.7	n/a	n/a

I

I Can't Believe It's Not Butter	Van Den Berghs	636	0.8	0.6	70.0	nil
light	Van Den Berghs	375	3.0	0.8	40.0	nil
Ice Cream						
dairy, vanilla		194	3.6	24.4	9.8	Tr
dairy, flavoured		179	3.5	24.7	8.0	Tr
non-dairy, vanilla		178	3.2	23.1	8.7	Tr
non-dairy, flavoured		166	3.1	23.2	7.4	Tr
mixes		182	4.1	25.1	7.9	Tr
Ice Cream Wafers		342	10.1	78.8	0.7	N
Iced Gem	Jacob's	394	5.2	86.2	3.1	1.4
Iced Tarts	Lyons Bakeries	445	3.3	71.8	16.0	1.1
Ice Magic, all flavours, as sold	Bird's	66.0	4.4	35.0	56.0	0.7

All amounts given per 100g/100ml unless otherwise stated

Product	*Brand*	*Calories kcal*	*Protein (g)*	*Carbo-hydrate (g)*	*Fat (g)*	*Dietary Fibre (g)*
Icing Sugar	Tate & Lyle	398	nil	99.6	nil	nil
Ideal Sauce	Heinz Ploughman's	109	0.6	26.4	0.1	0.5
Indian Chevda	Sharwood	523	7.1	44.3	36.5	7.2
Indian Chicken Stir Fry Meal	Ross	74.0	5.8	15.2	0.6	3.7
Indian Cuisine Madras Curry	Holland & Barrett	79.0	1.7	7.9	4.7	1.3
Indian Curry & Vegetables Stir Fry Sauce	Uncle Ben's	74.0	1.0	13.3	1.9	n/a
Indian Korma Cooking Sauce	Heinz Weight Watchers	49.0	1.5	8.2	0.8	1.0
Indian Oxo Cubes, each, as sold	Brooke Bond	21.0	0.7	3.4	0.5	n/a
Indian Special Fried Savoury Rice	Batchelors	517	11.8	10.3	7.0	1.8

Indian Special Rice	Ross	118	2.8	26.1	0.8	1.3
Indian Tandoori Prawns Stir Fry	Ross	67.0	3.8	11.6	1.6	2.1
Indian Tikka Masala	Campbell's	127	2.2	9.9	8.8	n/a
Indian Tikka Masala Cooking Sauce	Heinz Weight Watchers	48.0	1.5	6.8	1.6	0.5
Indonesian Nasi Goreng	Heinz Weight Watchers	89.0	6.3	11.0	2.2	0.7
Indonesian Satay Cook-In-Sauce	Homepride	180	5.5	12.6	12.0	n/a
Inspirations	Cadbury	500	6.1	55.6	28.0	n/a
Instant Coffee: ***see Coffee***						
Instant Creamy Mashed Potatoes, made up	Yeoman	60.0	1.6	12.9	0.2	n/a
Instant Dessert Powder		391	2.4	60.1	17.3	1.0
made up with whole milk		111	3.1	14.8	6.3	0.2
made up with skimmed milk		84.0	3.1	14.9	3.2	0.2

Product	*Brand*	*Calories kcal*	*Protein (g)*	*Carbo-hydrate (g)*	*Fat (g)*	*Dietary Fibre (g)*
Instant Milk: *see brands*						
Instant Potato Powder						
made up with water		57.0	1.5	13.5	0.1	1.0
made up with whole milk		76.0	2.4	14.8	1.2	1.0
made up with semi-skimmed milk		70.0	2.4	14.8	1.2	1.0
made up with skimmed milk		66.0	2.4	14.8	0.1	1.0
Instant Soup Powder, dried		341	6.5	64.4	14.0	N
made up with water		55.0	1.1	10.5	2.3	N
Irish Stew		123	5.3	9.1	7.6	0.9
	Tyne Brand	89.0	4.3	9.4	3.8	n/a
Irn Bru	Barr	43.0	n/a	10.6	Tr	Tr
diet	Barr	4.1	n/a	0.9	Tr	Tr
Italian Beans	Heinz	91.0	4.8	15.0	1.3	4.1
Italian Bean Salad	Batchelors	101	7.3	20.1	0.6	3.5
Italian Bolognese Sauce	Buitoni	60.0	3.3	9.1	0.9	0.3
Italian Chicken Pot Light	Golden Wonder	325	15.9	60.1	2.1	n/a

Italian Herbs & Garlic Pasta 'n' Sauce, as served	Batchelors	428	20.3	74.5	5.6	9.0
Italian Mince with Pasta, per pack	Birds Eye Menu Master	355	18.0	39.0	14.0	2.9
Italian Oxo Cubes, each, as sold	Brooke Bond	21.0	0.7	3.4	0.6	n/a
Italian Rice & Things Dry Mix, as sold	Crosse & Blackwell	370	8.7	75.4	3.4	2.6
Italian Style Chicken & Fresh Basil Sandwiches, per pack	Boots Shapers	194	n/a	n/a	n/a	n/a
Italian Supernoodles, per packet, as served	Batchelors	525	9.0	66.8	24.6	4.7
Italian Tomato & Onion Cooking Sauce	Heinz Weight Watchers	38.0	1.5	7.4	0.2	1.0
Italian Veg. Ragu Sauce	Batchelors	54.0	1.7	11.3	0.1	n/a
Italian Vinaigrette Maker	Lea & Perrins	90.0	0.5	20.0	0.2	n/a

All amounts given per 100g/100ml unless otherwise stated

J

Product	*Brand*	*Calories kcal*	*Protein (g)*	*Carbo-hydrate (g)*	*Fat (g)*	*Dietary Fibre (g)*
Jacket Potato Cheese & Onion, half	Birds Eye Country Club	180	6.0	23.0	8.0	n/a
Jacket Scallopes	Ross	127	2.9	21.2	3.4	1.8
Jackfruit, raw		88.0	1.3	21.4	0.3	N
canned, drained		104	0.5	26.3	0.3	N
Jaffa Cake Bars, each	Mr Kipling	164	2.1	25.2	5.8	n/a
Jaffa Cakes	McVitie's	376	3.9	72.3	8.2	0.9
Jaffa Fingers, each	Mr Kipling	136	0.8	17.7	6.9	n/a
Jaggery		367	0.5	97.2	nil	nil
Jalapeno Pepper Sauce	Lea & Perrins	94.0	0.6	21.7	0.5	n/a

Jalapeno Pepper with New York Cheddar Partner, 28g/1oz	Kavli	117	n/a	n/a	n/a	n/a
Jalfrezi Cook-In-Sauce	Homepride	66.0	1.4	10.3	2.3	n/a
Jam						
fruit with edible seeds		261	0.6	69.0	nil	N
stone fruit		261	0.4	69.3	nil	N
reduced sugar		123	0.5	31.9	0.1	N
Jam Doughnuts: *see Doughnuts*						
Jam Roly Poly	McVitie's	391	5.1	51.6	18.7	1.2
Jam Swiss Roll	Mr Kipling	211	2.5	48.1	2.3	n/a
Jam Tarts, recipe		380	3.3	62.0	14.9	1.6
retail		368	3.3	63.4	13.0	N
assorted	Lyons Bakeries	392	3.7	59.5	15.5	1.4
each	Mr Kipling	130	1.2	20.4	4.9	n/a
Jamaica Ginger Bar Cake	McVitie's	380	4.1	55.8	14.8	0.9
Jamaican Cook-In-Sauce	Homepride	99.0	1.1	11.5	5.4	n/a

Product	Brand	Calories kcal	Protein (g)	Carbo-hydrate (g)	Fat (g)	Dietary Fibre (g)
Japanese Beef Oriental Stir Fry	Ross	62.0	5.4	9.4	1.0	1.5
Japanese Noodles & Prawn Soup of the World	Knorr	298	13.6	53.3	3.4	n/a
Japanese Rice Crackers	Holland & Barrett	400	9.4	79.0	5.2	0.5
Jelly, made with water		61.0	1.2	15.1	nil	nil
Jelly Crystals: *see individual flavours*						
Jellytots	Nestlé	347	0.1	86.6	nil	n/a
Juicy Fruit Chewing Gum	Wrigley	304	nil	74.0	nil	nil

K

Kale: ***see Curly Kale***						
Kashmiri Chicken Curry	Findus Lean Cuisine	110	7.0	14.7	2.6	1.6
Kashmir Mild Curry Sauce	Colman's	80.0	0.8	n/a	4.9	n/a
Kashmir Mild Curry Sauce Mix	Sharwood	242	10.3	29.0	9.4	16.4
Kedgeree		166	14.2	10.5	7.9	Tr
Keema Curry with Cumin Rice Big Deal	Heinz Weight Watchers	94.0	5.1	12.2	2.7	0.5
Keg Bitter: ***see Beer***						
Ketchup, tomato		98.0	2.1	24.0	Tr	0.9

Product	*Brand*	*Calories kcal*	*Protein (g)*	*Carbo-hydrate (g)*	*Fat (g)*	*Dietary Fibre (g)*
Kidney						
lamb, fried		155	24.6	nil	6.3	nil
ox, stewed		172	25.6	nil	7.7	nil
pig, stewed		153	24.4	nil	6.1	nil
Kidney Beans: *see Red Kidney Beans*						
King Banana, each	Lyons Maid	140	0.8	12.0	9.9	n/a
King Cones (Lyons Maid): *see individual flavours*						
King Size Sausage Rolls	Kraft	320	6.6	24.7	22.3	n/a
Kingsmill White Bread	Allied Bakeries	233	8.6	45.1	2.0	2.3
Kingsmill White Rolls, each	Allied Bakeries	151	4.6	25.8	3.2	1.0
Kingsmill Wholemeal & Wheatgerm Bread	Allied Bakeries	217	10.7	36.9	2.9	6.0
Kipper Fillets with Butter	Birds Eye Captain's Table	220	17.5	nil	16.6	nil
Kippers, baked, flesh only		205	25.5	nil	11.4	nil

Kit Kat	Nestlé	501	7.4	59.4	26.0	n/a
Kiwi & Lime Spring, per pack	Boots Shapers	3.0	n/a	n/a	Tr	n/a
Kiwi Fruit		49.0	1.1	10.6	0.5	1.9
Kiwi Fruit in Syrup	Libby	69.0	n/a	n/a	Tr	n/a
Kohl Rabi, raw		23.0	1.6	3.7	0.2	2.2
boiled		18.0	1.2	3.1	0.2	1.9
Kola Chew Bar, each	Trebor Bassett	115	nil	24.7	1.7	nil
Kola Cubes	Cravens	386	Tr	96.4	nil	nil
each	Trebor Bassett	18.0	nil	4.4	nil	nil
Korma Classic Curry Sauce	Homepride	81.0	1.3	10.5	3.6	n/a
Korma Curry Sauce	Sharwood	88.0	2.2	8.5	5.0	2.3
Korma Mild Curry Sauce	Colman's	73.0	2.5	n/a	4.5	n/a
Krackawheat	McVitie's	518	8.3	61.0	25.8	4.9
Krona 70% Fat Spread	Van Den Berghs	638	0.3	1.9	70.0	nil
Krona Reduced Fat Spread	Van Den Berghs	548	0.3	1.8	60.0	nil

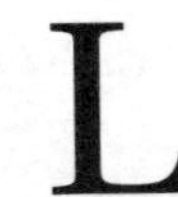

Product	Brand	Calories kcal	Protein (g)	Carbo-hydrate (g)	Fat (g)	Dietary Fibre (g)
Lady's Fingers: *see Okra*						
Lager, bottled		29.0	0.2	1.5	Tr	nil
Lamb, breast						
lean & fat, roast		410	19.1	nil	37.1	nil
lean only, roast		252	25.6	nil	16.6	nil
Lamb, chops						
loin, lean & fat, grilled		355	23.5	nil	29.0	nil
loin, lean only, grilled		222	27.8	nil	12.3	nil
Lamb, cutlets						
lean & fat, grilled		370	23.0	nil	30.9	nil
lean only, grilled		222	27.8	nil	12.3	nil
Lamb, leg						

lean & fat, roast		266	26.1	nil	17.9	nil
lean only, roast		191	29.4	nil	8.1	nil
Lamb, scrag & neck						
lean & fat, stewed		292	25.6	nil	21.1	nil
lean only, stewed		253	27.8	nil	15.7	nil
Lamb, shoulder						
lean & fat, roast		316	19.9	nil	26.3	nil
lean only, roast		196	23.8	nil	11.2	nil
Lamb & Vegetable Casserole	Heinz Lunch Bowl	86.0	5.0	8.3	3.7	1.4
Lamb Curry	Tyne Brand	99.0	6.1	7.2	5.1	n/a
Lamb Grillsteak, each	Birds Eye Steakhouse	175	14.0	1.0	13.0	nil
Lamb Hotpot Casserole Mix, as sold	Colman's	280	9.1	57.0	1.5	n/a
Lambourn Scooples, Original, each	Kavli	23.0	n/a	n/a	n/a	n/a

All amounts given per 100g/100ml unless otherwise stated

Product	*Brand*	*Calories kcal*	*Protein (g)*	*Carbo-hydrate (g)*	*Fat (g)*	*Dietary Fibre (g)*
Lamb Ragout Simply Fix Dry Mix, as sold	Crosse & Blackwell	345	10.6	59.5	7.3	2.2
Lamb Stock Cubes	Knorr	325	11.4	25.3	19.8	n/a
Lamb Tikka Masala	Findus Lean Cuisine	112	8.0	14.4	2.5	1.7
Lancashire Cheese		373	23.3	0.1	31.0	nil
Lancashire Hotpot	Tyne Brand	77.0	4.5	7.2	3.3	n/a
Lard		891	Tr	Tr	99.0	nil
Large Prunes	Holland & Barrett	134	2.0	33.5	Tr	13.4
Lasagne, frozen, cooked		102	5.0	12.8	3.8	N
	Findus Dinner Supreme	120	7.0	10.9	5.4	0.9
per pack	Birds Eye Menu Master	460	26.0	40.0	22.0	2.1
Lasagne (pasta), raw						

egg	Buitoni	342	13.4	68.0	1.8	3.5
standard	Buitoni	348	13.0	70.0	1.8	3.4
Lasagne Bolognese Ready Meal	Dolmio	132	7.0	11.7	6.3	n/a
Lasagne Microchef Meal	Batchelors	143	6.9	12.4	7.6	n/a
Lasagne Vegetale Ready Meal	Dolmio	101	3.0	11.6	4.7	n/a
Lasagne Verdi	Findus Lean Cuisine	84.0	7.1	9.2	2.1	1.2
Lattice Oven Fries	McCain	210	2.0	31.8	9.2	n/a
Lavash	International Harvest	281	10.4	56.3	1.6	5.5
Lean Beef Lasagne	Findus Lean Cuisine	91.0	6.2	11.5	2.2	1.1
per pack	Birds Eye Healthy Options	335	25.0	43.0	7.0	3.6
Lean Cuisine (Findus): ***see individual flavours***						

Product	*Brand*	*Calories kcal*	*Protein (g)*	*Carbo-hydrate (g)*	*Fat (g)*	*Dietary Fibre (g)*
Leek & Potato Quick Serve Soup, as served	Batchelors	320	3.6	47.7	13.4	n/a
Leek & Potato Slim-A-Soup Special, per sachet	Batchelors	59.0	1.1	11.0	1.5	n/a
Leek & Potato Soup	Batchelors	47.0	1.1	3.8	3.0	n/a
Leeks, boiled		21.0	1.2	2.6	0.7	1.7
Leicester Cheese		401	24.3	0.1	33.7	nil
Lemonade, bottled		21.0	Tr	5.6	nil	nil
	Barr	30.0	n/a	7.4	Tr	Tr
	Corona	10.0	Tr	2.3	nil	n/a
	R Whites	20.0	nil	5.4	Tr	n/a
low calorie	Barr	0.9	n/a	Tr	Tr	Tr
	Corona	0.5	n/a	nil	n/a	n/a
	R Whites	0.5	n/a	nil	n/a	n/a
Lemonade Shandy	Top Deck	24.0	Tr	6.4	Tr	n/a
Lemon & Ginger Sauce &						

Vegetables Stir Fry	Uncle Ben's	61.0	0.6	13.0	0.6	n/a
Lemon & Lime Crush, per pack	Boots Shapers	7.0	n/a	n/a	Tr	n/a
Lemon & Lime Drink	Jusoda	28.0	n/a	6.9	Tr	Tr
diluted	Quosh	29.0	n/a	7.6	n/a	n/a
no added sugar, diluted	Robinsons	11.0	0.1	0.7	Tr	n/a
ready to drink	Quosh	15.0	Tr	3.3	Tr	n/a
Lemon & Lime Glucose Energy Tablets	Lucozade Sport	339	Tr	90.4	n/a	n/a
Lemon & Lime Layered Desert, per pack	Boots Shapers	83.0	n/a	n/a	2.6	n/a
Lemon & Lime Yogurt Mousse, per pack	Boots Shapers	54.0	n/a	n/a	1.4	n/a
Lemon & Sultana Devonshire Cheesecake	St Ivel	276	6.7	29.8	15.2	n/a
Lemon Bakewells, each	Mr Kipling	204	2.1	30.9	8.8	n/a

All amounts given per 100g/100ml unless otherwise stated

Product	*Brand*	*Calories kcal*	*Protein (g)*	*Carbo-hydrate (g)*	*Fat (g)*	*Dietary Fibre (g)*
Lemon Barley Water, diluted	Quosh	20.0	Tr	4.7	Tr	n/a
	Robinsons	84.0	0.3	19.0	Tr	n/a
Lemon Cheesecake Mix	Green's/ Homepride	298	4.0	34.5	16.0	n/a
Lemon Chicken Stir Fry Dry Mix, as sold	Crosse & Blackwell	370	2.7	80.9	3.9	0.1
Lemon Curd Starch Base		283	0.6	62.7	5.1	0.2
Lemon Curd Tarts	Lyons Bakeries	416	3.5	61.8	17.2	1.0
Lemon Delight, per pack	Boots Shapers	116	n/a	n/a	3.9	n/a
Lemon Dessert Bombes	Heinz Weight Watchers	128	1.8	24.9	2.1	5.3
Lemon Drink	Tango	49.0	Tr	11.6	Tr	n/a
diluted	Quosh	20.0	n/a	5.2	n/a	n/a
low calorie	Tango	4.0	Tr	0.2	Tr	n/a
no added sugar, diluted	Robinsons	9.8	0.1	0.1	Tr	n/a

sparkling	St Clements	47.0	Tr	11.3	Tr	Tr
Lemon Flavour Jelly Crystals	Dietade	7.0	1.5	0.1	nil	nil
Lemon Iced Gingerbread	California Cake & Cookie Ltd	291	5.7	48.5	9.6	1.1
Lemon Iced Slices	Lyons Bakeries	390	3.7	61.4	14.4	0.8
Lemon Juice, fresh		7.0	0.3	1.6	Tr	0.1
Lemon Juice Drink	Citrus Spring	38.0	Tr	10.0	Tr	n/a
Lemon Low Calorie Squash	Dietade	7.0	nil	0.4	nil	n/a
Lemon Matchmakers	Nestlé	476	5.1	68.8	20.2	n/a
Lemon Meringue Crunch Mix	Green's/ Homepride	249	2.5	39.0	9.0	n/a
Lemon Meringue Gateau	McVitie's	276	4.5	25.8	17.9	Tr
Lemon Meringue Pie, recipe		319	4.5	45.9	14.4	0.7
Lemon Meringue Premium Ice Cream	Heinz Weight Watchers	159	3.1	25.8	4.4	nil

Product	*Brand*	*Calories kcal*	*Protein (g)*	*Carbo-hydrate (g)*	*Fat (g)*	*Dietary Fibre (g)*
Lemon, Orange, Hazelnut & Raisin Yogurt, low fat	Holland & Barrett	105	5.4	17.3	1.6	0.2
Lemon Puff	Jacob's	531	5.3	59.1	30.3	1.4
Lemon Rice	Sharwood	358	7.5	71.9	3.2	1.3
Lemons, whole, without pips		19.0	1.0	3.2	0.3	N
Lemon Slices, each	Mr Kipling	125	1.1	18.8	4.9	n/a
Lemon Sole						
fried in crumbs		216	16.1	9.3	13.0	0.4
steamed		91.0	20.6	nil	0.9	nil
Lemon Sorbet		131	0.9	34.2	Tr	nil
	Fiesta	114	nil	28.1	nil	n/a
Lemon Sponge Pudding	Heinz	308	2.8	49.7	10.9	0.6
Lemon Toppit, each	Nestlé	90.0	1.3	18.4	1.2	n/a
Lemon Whole Fruit Drink, diluted	Robinsons	76.0	0.1	18.0	Tr	n/a

Lentil & Bacon Cup-A-Soup Special, per sachet	Batchelors	89.0	3.4	14.3	2.4	n/a
Lentil & Bacon Soup	Baxters	56.0	2.0	7.6	1.0	0.9
Lentil & Carrot Soup	Heinz Weight Watchers	26.0	1.3	5.0	0.1	0.4
Lentil & Chicken Wholesome Soup	Heinz Weight Watchers	32.0	1.8	5.4	0.4	1.0
Lentil & Vegetable Soup	Baxters	34.0	1.9	6.8	0.1	1.5
Lentil Dhal	Holland & Barrett	89.0	4.1	9.5	4.0	1.7
Lentils						
green/brown, boiled		105	8.8	16.9	0.7	3.8
red, boiled		100	7.6	17.5	0.4	1.9
Lentil Soup		99.0	4.4	12.7	3.8	1.1
	Campbell's	46.0	2.5	7.4	0.6	n/a
	Heinz Wholesoup	36.0	2.2	6.4	nil	0.9

All amounts given per 100g/100ml unless otherwise stated

Product	*Brand*	*Calories kcal*	*Protein (g)*	*Carbo-hydrate (g)*	*Fat (g)*	*Dietary Fibre (g)*
Lettuce, average, raw		14.0	0.8	1.7	0.5	0.9
Light 'n' Tasty Sausage Rolls	Kraft	266	8.1	24.5	15.8	n/a
Light Brown Soft Sugar	Tate & Lyle	386	0.1	95.8	nil	nil
Light Cheese Singles, each	Primula	45.0	n/a	n/a	n/a	n/a
Lightly Salted Crisps, per pack	Boots Shapers	96.0	n/a	n/a	4.8	n/a
Lightly Salted Golden Lights, per pack	Golden Wonder	98.0	1.0	13.8	4.3	0.6
Light Reduced Calorie Mayonnaise	Hellmanns	300	0.7	2.3	29.8	n/a
Light Soy Chinese Pouring Sauce	Sharwood	18.0	4.4	0.2	Tr	0.3
Light Spreadable Cheddar, 28g/1oz	Primula	69.0	n/a	n/a	n/a	n/a

with Chives & Onion, 28g/1oz	Primula	71.0	n/a	n/a	n/a	n/a
with Ham & Mustard, 28g/1oz	Primula	71.0	n/a	n/a	n/a	n/a
Lima Beans: *see Butter Beans*						
Limeade & Lager	Top Deck	27.0	Tr	6.4	Tr	n/a
Limeade, bottles	Corona	8.0	Tr	1.9	nil	n/a
Limeade, cans	Corona	23.0	nil	6.0	nil	n/a
Lime Cordial, diluted	Britvic	17.0	Tr	4.6	Tr	n/a
	Quosh	18.0	n/a	4.8	n/a	n/a
Lime Crusha	Burgess	123	nil	30.6	nil	nil
Lime Flavour Cordial, diluted	Quosh	8.0	Tr	1.5	Tr	n/a
Lime Juice Cordial, undiluted		112	Tr	27.0	nil	nil
diluted	Robinsons	83.0	0.1	19.0	Tr	n/a
Lime Juice Drink	Citrus Spring	45.0	Tr	10.6	Tr	n/a
Lime Pickle	Sharwood	152	2.6	2.1	3.6	3.3

All amounts given per 100g/100ml unless otherwise stated

Product	*Brand*	*Calories kcal*	*Protein (g)*	*Carbo-hydrate (g)*	*Fat (g)*	*Dietary Fibre (g)*
Lincoln Biscuits	McVitie's	508	5.8	67.1	23.5	2.0
Linguine	Napolina	320	11.5	68.4	1.5	5.6
Lion Bar	Nestlé	477	5.5	62.9	22.6	n/a
Lion Bar Ice Cream, each	Nestlé	227	3.4	23.6	13.3	n/a
Lip Smacker, each	Lyons Maid	77.0	nil	19.4	nil	n/a
Liqueur Gateau	Mr Kipling	428	5.1	54.4	17.9	n/a
Liquorice Allsorts		313	3.9	74.1	2.2	N
Liquorice Toffees	Itona	395	0.6	66.5	15.2	n/a
Liquorice Torpedoes, each	Trebor Bassett	5.1	nil	1.2	nil	nil
Liver						
calf, fried		254	26.9	7.3	13.2	0.2
chicken, fried		194	20.7	3.4	10.9	0.2
lamb, fried		232	22.9	3.9	14.0	0.1
ox, stewed		198	24.8	3.6	9.5	Tr
pig, stewed		189	25.6	3.6	8.1	Tr

Food	Brand					
Liver & Bacon Casserole Cooking Mix, as sold	Colman's	289	10.0	58.0	1.2	n/a
Liver & Bacon Pâté	Shippams	187	17.0	1.8	12.4	n/a
Liver Pâté		316	13.1	1.0	28.9	Tr
low fat		191	18.0	2.8	12.0	Tr
Liver Sausage		310	12.9	4.3	26.9	0.5
Liver with Onions & Gravy, per pack	Birds Eye Menu Master	154	16.0	5.0	6.0	0.5
Lobster, boiled		119	22.1	nil	3.4	nil
	Young's	119	22.1	nil	3.4	nil
Lobster Bisque	Baxters	54.0	6.5	5.2	2.1	0.2
Lockets	Mars	383	nil	95.8	nil	n/a
Long Grain & Wild Rice, as sold	Uncle Ben's	347	11.2	92.8	1.2	n/a
Long Grain Rice, as sold	Uncle Ben's	342	7.8	75.4	1.0	n/a
	Whitworths	361	6.5	86.8	1.0	0.5
frozen	Uncle Ben's	140	3.0	30.3	0.7	n/a
3 min	Uncle Ben's	127	2.7	27.3	0.8	n/a

All amounts given per 100g/100ml unless otherwise stated

Product	*Brand*	*Calories kcal*	*Protein (g)*	*Carbo-hydrate (g)*	*Fat (g)*	*Dietary Fibre (g)*
Low Fat Apricot, Guava & Banana Yogurt	Holland & Barrett	97.0	5.4	16.9	0.8	0.1
Low Fat Blackberry Yogurt	Holland & Barrett	84.0	5.4	13.8	0.8	n/a
Low Fat Dairy Spread						
with Cheese	Primula	46.0	n/a	n/a	n/a	n/a
with Cheese & Ham	Primula	46.0	n/a	n/a	n/a	n/a
with Cheese, Garlic & Herbs	Primula	175	20.0	4.0	9.0	n/a
with Ham	Primula	46.0	n/a	n/a	n/a	n/a
Low Fat Dressing	Heinz Weight Watchers	106	1.5	15.4	4.3	nil
Low Fat Spread		390	5.8	0.5	40.5	nil
Low Fat Strawberry & Red Cherry Yogurt	Holland & Barrett	97.0	6.4	16.9	0.8	0.1
Low Fat Strawberry Yogurt	Holland					

	& Barrett	83.0	5.4	13.4	0.8	0.2
Lucozade		67.0	Tr	18.0	nil	nil
light	SmithKline Beecham	37.0	Tr	9.1	nil	nil
Lucozade Orange Sport	SmithKline Beecham	28.0	Tr	6.4	nil	nil
Luncheon Meat, canned		313	12.6	5.5	26.9	0.3
Lunchpack & Brussels Pâté, per pack	Boots Shapers	202	n/a	n/a	8.8	n/a
Lunchpack & Cheese, per pack	Boots Shapers	148	n/a	n/a	2.7	n/a
Lunchpack & Cheese & Onion, per pack	Boots Shapers	149	n/a	n/a	2.7	n/a
Lunchpack & Provençal Pâté, per pack	Boots Shapers	198	n/a	n/a	8.0	n/a
Lunchpack with Cheese Spread & Crispbread Scoops, per pack	Boots Shapers	136	n/a	n/a	2.7	n/a

All amounts given per 100g/100ml unless otherwise stated

Product	*Brand*	*Calories kcal*	*Protein (g)*	*Carbo-hydrate (g)*	*Fat (g)*	*Dietary Fibre (g)*
Lunchpack with Dip & Mini Snacks, per pack	Boots Shapers	254	n/a	n/a	13.8	n/a
Luxury Raisin Country Crisp	Jordan's	424	3.7	32.3	8.2	4.0
Luxury Rum Xmas Pudding	Holland & Barrett	311	4.2	60.6	6.7	2.8
Luxury Wholemeal Xmas Pudding	Holland & Barrett	307	3.9	59.7	7.5	nil
Lychees						
raw		58.0	0.9	14.3	0.1	0.7
canned in syrup		68.0	0.4	17.7	Tr	0.5
	Libby	74.0	n/a	n/a	Tr	n/a

M

Food	Brand					
Macadamia Nuts, salted		748	7.9	4.8	77.6	5.3
Macaroni, boiled		86.0	3.0	18.5	0.5	0.9
Macaroni Cheese		178	7.3	13.6	10.8	0.5
	Findus Dinner Supreme	177	7.4	16.9	9.3	0.1
	Heinz	94.0	3.4	9.7	4.6	0.3
per pack	Birds Eye Menu Master	415	19.0	35.0	22.0	1.3
McChicken Sandwich, each	McDonald's	370	18.3	38.6	15.8	2.1
Mackerel, fried, flesh only		188	21.5	nil	11.3	nil
Madeira Cake		393	5.4	58.4	16.9	0.9
	Mr Kipling	325	4.6	47.1	14.5	n/a

All amounts given per 100g/100ml unless otherwise stated

Product	*Brand*	*Calories kcal*	*Protein (g)*	*Carbo-hydrate (g)*	*Fat (g)*	*Dietary Fibre (g)*
Madeira Loaf Mix	Green's	339	4.9	56.0	12.4	n/a
Madeira Wine Gravy Sauce Dry Mix, as sold	Crosse & Blackwell	358	8.4	63.1	8.0	1.5
Madras Classic Curry Sauce	Homepride	54.0	2.2	9.6	0.6	n/a
Madras Curry Sauce	Sharwood	100	1.7	6.9	7.3	1.6
Madras Medium Curry Casserole Mix, as sold	Colman's	281	6.4	51.0	5.0	n/a
Major Grey Chutney	Sharwood	215	0.4	52.9	0.2	1.0
Malaysian Chicken & Sweetcorn Soup of the World	Knorr	387	11.1	59.6	11.6	n/a
Malaysian Mild Curry Paste	Sharwood	252	5.2	9.9	21.1	6.6
Malt Bread		268	8.3	56.8	2.4	N
Malted Food Drink (Horlicks): ***see Horlicks***						

Maltesers	Mars	494	10.0	61.4	23.1	n/a
Malt Extract	Holland & Barrett	300	0.4	78.0	n/a	n/a
Maltlets Horlicks	SmithKline Beecham	384	12.4	78.0	4.0	n/a
Malt Vinegar	HP	4.6	Tr	1.1	nil	nil
Mandarin Delight, per pack	Boots Shapers	120	n/a	n/a	4.8	n/a
Mandarin Oranges						
canned in juice		32.0	0.7	7.7	Tr	0.3
	Libby	41.0	n/a	n/a	Tr	n/a
canned in syrup		52.0	0.5	14.4	Tr	0.2
	Libby	57.0	n/a	n/a	Tr	n/a
Mange-tout, raw		32.0	3.6	4.2	0.2	2.3
boiled		26.0	3.2	3.3	0.1	2.2
stir-fried		71.0	3.8	3.5	4.8	2.4
Mango & Apple Chutney	Sharwood	233	0.4	57.6	0.1	1.1
Mango & Chilli Pickle	Sharwood	83.0	2.0	3.4	5.9	3.4

All amounts given per 100g/100ml unless otherwise stated

Product	*Brand*	*Calories kcal*	*Protein (g)*	*Carbo-hydrate (g)*	*Fat (g)*	*Dietary Fibre (g)*
Mango & Lime Chutney	Sharwood	206	0.4	50.5	0.3	0.8
Mango Chutney, oily		285	0.4	49.5	10.9	0.9
Mango Chutney, Green Label	Sharwood	234	0.3	57.8	0.2	0.9
Mangoes						
ripe, raw, flesh only		57.0	0.7	14.1	0.2	2.6
canned in syrup		77.0	0.3	20.3	Tr	0.7
	Libby	70.0	n/a	n/a	Tr	n/a
Manor House Cake	Mr Kipling	513	5.3	57.7	29.0	n/a
Maple Cured Hickory Smoked Ham & Soft Cheese with Salad Bagel, each	Boots Shapers	199	n/a	n/a	n/a	n/a
Maple Flavour Pouring Syrup	Lyle's	284	Tr	76.0	nil	nil
Maple Walnut Cake	California Cake & Cookie Ltd	446	5.2	57.6	23.3	2.3
Maple Walnut Napoli	Lyons Maid	118	2.0	12.9	6.5	n/a

Margarine, average		739	0.2	1.0	81.6	nil
Margherita Ragu Pizza Topping	Batchelors	68.0	1.9	10.4	2.4	1.3
Marie Biscuits	Peek Frean	452	6.7	73.6	14.5	2.2
Marinara Ragu Pizza Topping	Batchelors	65.0	2.0	7.7	3.1	1.4
Marmalade		261	0.1	69.5	nil	0.6
reduced sugar	Holland & Barrett	140	0.5	36.0	nil	nil
sucrose free	Dietade	267	0.2	66.4	Tr	nil
Marmite		172	39.7	1.8	0.7	nil
Marrow						
raw, flesh only		12.0	0.5	2.2	0.2	0.5
boiled		9.0	0.4	1.6	0.2	0.6
Marrowfat Peas, canned		100	6.9	17.5	0.8	4.1
Mars Bar	Mars	452	4.0	69.6	17.5	n/a
Marzipan, homemade		461	10.4	50.2	25.8	3.3
retail		404	5.3	67.6	14.4	1.9

Product	*Brand*	*Calories kcal*	*Protein (g)*	*Carbo-hydrate (g)*	*Fat (g)*	*Dietary Fibre (g)*
Matchmakers: *see individual flavours*						
Matzo Crackers	Rakusen	335	10.8	76.7	0.4	5.7
Mayonnaise		691	1.1	1.7	75.6	nil
	Heinz	531	1.2	5.5	56.1	nil
light	Heinz Weight Watchers	265	0.9	7.2	25.9	nil
Meatballs & Beans	Campbell's	109	6.5	16.0	2.3	n/a
Meatballs in Chicken Gravy	Campbell's	119	6.2	8.4	6.9	n/a
Meatballs in Gravy	Campbell's	104	5.5	4.7	7.0	n/a
Meatballs in Onion Gravy	Campbell's	104	5.4	4.8	7.0	n/a
Meatballs in Tomato Sauce	Campbell's	113	5.6	7.0	6.9	n/a
Meat Paste		173	15.2	3.0	11.2	0.1
Mediterranean Chicken	Heinz Weight Watchers	87.0	6.0	10.6	2.2	0.6
Mediterranean Special Fried Savoury Rice	Batchelors	498	11.4	99.8	6.7	1.7

Mediterranean Tomato Sauce, as sold	Oxo	335	8.9	64.6	4.6	n/a
Mediterranean Tomato Slim-A-Soup, per sachet	Batchelors	38.0	1.1	8.3	0.3	n/a
Mediterranean Tomato Soup	Baxters	30.0	1.1	6.3	0.3	0.6
	Heinz Weight Watchers	26.0	0.5	4.3	0.7	0.7
Medium Curry Paste	Sharwood	369	4.3	14.0	32.8	6.9
Medium Egg Noodles	Sharwood	340	10.8	70.1	1.8	2.9
Medium Fat Soft Cheese		179	9.2	3.1	14.5	nil
Medium Hot Salsa	Heinz	30.0	1.7	5.5	0.2	1.4
Medium-Hot Salsa Style Ketchup	Heinz	78.0	2.2	17.0	0.2	1.6
Mega King Cone, each	Lyons Maid	367	6.2	46.4	18.7	n/a
Mega Mint King Cone, each	Lyons Maid	367	6.2	46.4	18.7	n/a
Mello Reduced Fat Spread	Kraft	540	0.3	1.0	60.0	nil
	Vitalite	540	0.3	1.0	60.0	nil

All amounts given per 100g/100ml unless otherwise stated

Product	Brand	Calories kcal	Protein (g)	Carbo-hydrate (g)	Fat (g)	Dietary Fibre (g)
Melon, flesh only						
Cantaloupe-type		19.0	0.6	4.2	0.1	1.0
Galia		24.0	0.5	5.6	0.1	0.4
Honeydew		28.0	0.6	6.6	0.1	0.6
Watermelon		31.0	0.5	7.1	0.3	0.1
Menu Master Meals (Birds Eye): *see individual flavours*						
Meringue		379	5.3	95.4	Tr	nil
Mexican Bean Salad	Batchelors	133	8.1	21.2	1.7	n/a
Mexican Cheese & Chilli Crisps, per pack	Golden Wonder	204	2.8	16.4	14.1	1.8
Mexican Chilli Rice & Things Dry Mix, as sold	Crosse & Blackwell	370	18.7	72.1	5.0	3.7
Mexican Chilli Sauce	Campbell's	73.0	3.9	13.3	0.5	n/a
Mexican Chilli with Kidney Beans Cooking Sauce	Heinz Weight Watchers	40.0	1.7	7.1	0.5	1.1
Mexican Chilli with Rice	Heinz Weight Watchers	90.0	5.8	12.7	1.8	0.9

Mexican Extra Hot Chilli Sauce	Homepride	52.0	1.3	10.8	0.4	n/a
Mexican Hot Chilli Sauce	Homepride	54.0	1.3	11.0	0.6	n/a
Mexican Medium Chilli Sauce	Homepride	52.0	1.2	10.9	0.4	n/a
Mexican Mild Chilli Sauce	Homepride	52.0	1.2	10.9	0.4	n/a
Mexican Special Fried Savoury Rice, per packet, as served	Batchelors	498	11.4	99.8	6.7	6.2
Mexican Spicy Barbecue Sauce	Lea & Perrins	115	1.4	25.2	0.9	n/a
Mexican Spicy Tomato & Bacon Soup of the World	Knorr	307	8.8	59.5	3.7	n/a
Mexican Spicy Tomato Cup-A-Soup, per sachet	Batchelors	80.0	1.5	17.7	0.9	n/a
Mexicorn	Green Giant	80.0	2.4	17.5	0.5	3.7
Mickey, each	Lyons Maid	98.0	2.2	11.7	4.7	n/a
Microchef Meals & Snacks (Batchelors): ***see individual flavours***						

Product	Brand	Calories kcal	Protein (g)	Carbo-hydrate (g)	Fat (g)	Dietary Fibre (g)
Midnight Hot Chocolate, per pack	Boots Shapers	40.0	n/a	n/a	0.9	n/a
Midnight Mint Class	Jacob's	520	4.1	58.7	29.9	2.1
Midnight Orange Club Class	Jacob's	516	4.2	61.3	28.2	2.1
Mighty Munchers, each	Allied Bakeries	210	7.6	35.2	4.4	2.0
Mighty White Bread	Allied Bakeries	227	7.7	45.6	1.5	3.1
Mildbake Brown Bread	Hovis	217	8.7	41.8	1.7	4.7
Mild Beer: ***see Beer***						
Mild Cheese & Broccoli Pasta 'n' Sauce, as served	Batchelors	513	24.1	97.2	6.8	9.5
Mild Cheese Rice & Things Dry Mix, as sold	Crosse & Blackwell	380	10.9	71.7	5.2	2.1
Mild Curry Beanfeast, per packet, as served	Batchelors	406	5.3	65.2	6.7	n/a
Mild Curry Paste	Sharwood	356	4.8	4.8	35.3	7.1

Mild Curry Rice & Things Dry Mix, as sold	Crosse & Blackwell	350	7.9	69.2	4.5	3.3
Mild Curry Savoury Rice, per packet, as served	Batchelors	467	8.4	97.1	5.0	6.0
Mild Curry Supernoodles, per packet, as served	Batchelors	520	9.1	65.6	24.5	4.7
Mild Indian Curry Sauce, as sold	Oxo	383	11.1	62.5	9.8	n/a
Mild Kashmiri Curry Sauce Dry Mix, as sold	Crosse & Blackwell	379	12.8	52.0	13.3	3.4
Mild-Medium Hot Salsa	Heinz	29.0	1.6	5.3	0.2	1.3
Mild-Medium Salsa Style Ketchup	Heinz	78.0	2.2	16.8	0.2	1.6
Mild Mustard Low Fat Dressing	Heinz Weight Watchers	62.0	2.0	5.4	3.6	nil
Mild Mustard Pickle	Heinz Ploughman's	128	2.4	26.7	1.3	1.0

All amounts given per 100g/100ml unless otherwise stated

Product	*Brand*	*Calories kcal*	*Protein (g)*	*Carbo-hydrate (g)*	*Fat (g)*	*Dietary Fibre (g)*
Mild Veg. Curry	Holland & Barrett	86.0	1.5	8.0	5.6	1.3
Mild Vegetable Curry	Sharwood	66.0	1.5	4.9	4.5	1.0
Milk (see also condensed, soya, etc.)						
semi-skimmed, average		46.0	3.3	5.0	1.6	nil
skimmed, average		33.0	3.3	5.0	0.1	nil
whole, average		66.0	3.2	4.8	3.9	nil
Milk & Plain Chocolate Caramels	Cravens	493	Tr	96.4	nil	nil
Milk Chocolate		529	8.4	59.4	30.3	Tr
	Nestlé	520	7.4	60.3	29.5	n/a
Milk Chocolate Aero	Nestlé	523	8.3	55.1	29.9	n/a
Milk Chocolate Breakaway	Nestlé	538	7.7	62.9	28.4	n/a
Milk Chocolate Cake Bars	Mr Kipling	173	2.4	21.0	8.4	n/a
Milk Chocolate Dessert Pot	Ambrosia	119	3.4	19.7	3.0	n/a

Milk Chocolate Finger Biscuits	Cadbury	515	6.9	66.1	24.9	n/a
Milk Chocolate Mousse, per pack	Boots Shapers	88.0	n/a	n/a	2.8	n/a
Milk Chocolate Multipack, per pack	Boots Shapers	198	n/a	n/a	4.5	n/a
Milk Chocolate Wafers	Cadbury	537	6.4	61.6	29.4	n/a
Milk Chocolate Yorkie	Nestlé	525	7.0	58.1	29.4	n/a
Milk Classico, each	Lyons Maid	141	1.7	13.5	9.0	n/a
Milk Pudding						
made with whole milk		129	3.9	19.9	4.3	0.1
made with semi-skimmed milk		93.0	4.0	20.1	0.2	0.1
Milk Stick, each	Nestlé	275	3.5	23.6	18.5	n/a
Milk Tray	Cadbury	480	5.1	62.7	23.3	n/a
Milky Bar/Buttons	Nestlé	549	8.4	55.6	32.5	n/a
Milky Bar Dessert	Chambourcy	253	4.8	22.0	16.2	nil

All amounts given per 100g/100ml unless otherwise stated

Product	*Brand*	*Calories kcal*	*Protein (g)*	*Carbo-hydrate (g)*	*Fat (g)*	*Dietary Fibre (g)*
Milkybar Ice Cream, each	Nestlé	114	2.0	9.6	7.5	n/a
Milky Way	Mars	454	4.2	72.0	16.6	n/a
Millionaires Shortbread	California Cake & Cookie Ltd	383	6.9	58.0	25.1	n/a
Mince & Brandy Sauce Pies, each	Mr Kipling	284	2.7	40.8	10.9	n/a
Mince & Onion Beanfeast, per packet, as served	Batchelors	356	30.3	50.2	5.2	n/a
Mince, Beans & Barbecue Sauce	Tyne Brand	109	8.1	11.6	3.4	n/a
Mince Bolognese	Tyne Brand	116	10.2	4.7	6.3	n/a
Minced Beef: *see Beef*						
Minced Beef & Onion	Tyne Brand	115	9.5	7.0	5.5	n/a
Minced Beef & Onion Deep Pie	Ross	249	6.0	24.6	14.5	1.0

Minced Beef & Onion Pie	Ross	295	6.6	24.6	19.4	1.0
	Tyne Brand	161	8.7	13.3	8.1	n/a
Minced Beef Crispy Pancakes	Findus	168	7.2	23.0	5.2	1.0
Minced Beef with Vegetables & Gravy, per pack	Birds Eye Menu Master	155	16.0	9.0	6.0	1.0
Minced Beef with Vegetables & Potato, per pack	Birds Eye Menu Master	380	18.0	36.0	18.0	3.1
Mincemeat		274	0.6	62.1	4.3	1.3
Mince, Pasta & Tomato Sauce	Tyne Brand	117	7.8	9.3	5.4	n/a
Mince Pies	Holland & Barrett	317	3.8	53.7	16.0	4.2
each	Mr Kipling	244	2.1	39.0	8.8	n/a
Minestrone Cup-A-Soup Special, per sachet	Batchelors	79.0	1.3	15.2	1.9	n/a
Minestrone Low Calorie Soup	Knorr	301	11.0	62.8	0.6	n/a
Minestrone Packet Soup, as served	Batchelors	218	6.0	48.1	1.9	3.9

All amounts given per 100g/100ml unless otherwise stated

Product	Brand	Calories kcal	Protein (g)	Carbo-hydrate (g)	Fat (g)	Dietary Fibre (g)
Minestrone Slim-A-Soup Special, per sachet	Batchelors	57.0	1.4	10.2	0.6	n/a
Minestrone Soup, canned	Baxters	30.0	1.3	6.0	0.2	1.0
	Heinz	32.0	1.4	4.7	0.8	0.6
	Heinz Weight Watchers	18.0	0.7	3.1	0.3	0.5
Minestrone Soup, dried						
as served		23.0	0.8	3.7	8.8	N
as sold		298	10.1	47.6	8.8	N
Minestrone with Pasta Soup	Batchelors	25.0	1.4	4.8	0.1	n/a
Mini Crispbread, per pack	Boots Shapers	68.0	n/a	n/a	0.5	n/a
Mini Logs	Mr Kipling	124	1.6	16.0	5.6	n/a
Mini Muesli Crispbreads, per pack	Boots Shapers	84.0	n/a	n/a	0.9	n/a
Mini Pizza Bases	Napolina	1189	8.5	55.8	4.1	n/a
Mini Ritz Crackers	Jacob's	523	6.5	57.5	29.7	2.1

Mini Yum Yums	Sunblest	422	4.4	54.3	20.8	1.0
Mint Aero	Nestlé	522	7.7	58.3	28.7	n/a
Mint Assortment	Cravens	414	0.3	89.4	6.1	nil
Mint Choc Chip King Cone, each	Lyons Maid	185	3.0	23.6	8.6	n/a
Mint Choc Chip Mousse, each	Fiesta	84.0	1.8	10.6	4.1	n/a
Mint Choc Chip Napoli	Lyons Maid	124	2.1	13.7	6.8	n/a
Mint Chocolate Dessert Bombes	Heinz Weight Watchers	126	2.3	23.9	2.4	6.2
Mint Club Biscuits	Jacob's	509	5.9	61.1	26.7	1.5
Mint Crisp, each	Lyons Maid	198	1.7	22.0	11.4	n/a
Minted Garden Peas	Ross	72.0	6.0	14.5	0.8	4.3
Mintetts	G. Payne & Co	415	6.1	91.0	3.0	n/a
Mint Humbugs	Cravens	413	0.6	89.7	5.8	nil
Minties	Nestlé	404	0.5	91.5	4.0	n/a

All amounts given per 100g/100ml unless otherwise stated

Product	*Brand*	*Calories kcal*	*Protein (g)*	*Carbo-hydrate (g)*	*Fat (g)*	*Dietary Fibre (g)*
Mint Imperials	Cravens	387	nil	96.3	nil	nil
each	Trebor Bassett	18.4	nil	4.6	nil	nil
Mint Jelly	Baxters	251	Tr	67.0	Tr	1.7
	Burgess	158	0.4	37.6	0.7	0.5
	Colman's	363	0.1	89.0	0.1	n/a
Mint Leaves	Cadbury	453	3.0	69.4	15.7	n/a
Mint Matchmakers	Nestlé	477	5.1	68.7	20.2	n/a
Mintola	Nestlé	430	3.4	67.3	16.4	n/a
Mints: *see individual types*						
Mint Sauce	Baxters	110	0.9	28.1	0.2	Tr
	Burgess	68.0	1.6	12.0	nil	2.0
	Colman's	122	0.8	26.0	0.1	n/a
	HP	156	2.1	26.1	1.8	n/a
Mint Toffees	Itona	360	0.6	67.0	11.0	n/a
Mint YoYo	McVitie's	523	4.7	63.9	27.7	0.8

Miracle Whip Dressing	Kraft	440	1.0	12.0	43.0	n/a
Miso		203	13.3	23.5	6.2	N
Mississippi Mud Pie	Green's/ Homepride	323	4.0	37.5	17.5	n/a
Mivvis (Lyons Maid): *see individual flavours*						
Mixed Bean Salad	Heinz	172	3.6	15.9	10.4	2.7
	Holland & Barrett	56.0	2.8	10.2	0.4	1.3
Mixed Berry Reduced Sugar Jam	Holland & Barrett	140	0.5	36.0	nil	nil
Mixed Fruit, dried		227	3.6	52.9	1.6	2.2
Mixed Fruit Sponge Pudding	Heinz	302	4.0	44.5	12.0	1.3
Mixed Fruit Sucrose Free Jam	Dietade	245	0.3	60.3	Tr	n/a
Mixed Nuts		607	22.9	7.9	54.1	6.0
Mixed Peel		231	0.3	59.1	0.9	4.8

Product	Brand	Calories kcal	Protein (g)	Carbo-hydrate (g)	Fat (g)	Dietary Fibre (g)
Mixed Peppers, dried	Whitworths	212	21.7	21.7	4.9	8.9
Mixed Peppers Rice & Things Dry Mix, as sold	Crosse & Blackwell	370	9.3	75.9	3.0	2.9
Mixed Vegetables						
frozen, boiled		42.0	3.3	6.6	0.5	N
canned		38.0	1.9	6.1	0.8	1.7
stir fry type, frozen, fried in oil		64.0	2.0	6.4	3.6	N
Mocha Hot Chocolate, per pack	Boots Shapers	40.0	n/a	n/a	0.9	n/a
Moghlai Chicken Korma Microwave Meal	Sharwood	162	7.0	17.0	7.8	1.4
Monkey Nuts: *see Peanuts*						
Mono Spread	St Ivel	675	nil	nil	75.0	nil
Montanara Ragu Cream Sauce	Batchelors	137	1.8	3.8	12.7	1.1
Mooli: *see Radish, white*						

Moonshine	Libby	48.0	Tr	12.0	Tr	nil
Morello Cherry Jam, reduced sugar	Heinz Weight Watchers	127	0.4	31.1	nil	0.4
Moussaka		184	9.1	7.0	13.6	0.9
	Findus Lean Cuisine	76.0	5.2	8.5	2.2	0.9
Moussaka Simply Fix Dry Mix, as sold	Crosse & Blackwell	330	8.9	48.3	11.0	7.7
Mousse: *see individual flavours*						
Mr Brain's Meals (Kraft): *see individual flavours*						
Muesli						
Swiss style		363	9.8	72.2	5.9	6.4
with no added sugar		366	10.5	67.1	7.8	7.6
Muesli Crispbread, 28g/1oz	Kavli	80.0	n/a	n/a	n/a	n/a
Muffins	Sunblest	226	8.2	45.9	1.1	2.4
Muffins with Cheese	Sunblest	221	8.4	40.2	2.9	1.4

All amounts given per 100g/100ml unless otherwise stated

Product	*Brand*	*Calories kcal*	*Protein (g)*	*Carbo-hydrate (g)*	*Fat (g)*	*Dietary Fibre (g)*
Mulligatawny Soup	Heinz	55.0	1.5	5.3	3.0	0.5
Multigrain Cob	Holland & Barrett	230	10.0	44.0	1.6	6.7
Multi-Grain Start	Kellogg's	370	7.0	79.0	2.5	5.0
Munchies	Nestlé	477	5.5	63.1	22.5	n/a
Munchmallows	McVitie's	448	5.3	70.0	16.5	1.1
Mung beans, boiled		91.0	7.6	15.3	0.4	4.8
Mung Beansprouts: *see Beansprouts*						
Murray Mints, each	Trebor Bassett	26.2	nil	5.7	0.3	nil
Mushroom A La Creme Pasta Choice Dry Mix, as sold	Crosse & Blackwell	400	17.0	60.2	10.4	2.6
Mushroom & Bacon Toast Topper	Heinz	93.0	6.9	6.5	4.4	0.3
Mushroom & Garlic Low In Fat Sauce	Homepride	293	1.1	7.6	3.9	n/a

Mushroom & Garlic Pizza	San Marco	241	11.3	28.5	10.4	1.2
Mushroom & Herb Soup	Batchelors	50.0	0.9	4.3	3.4	n/a
Mushroom & Pepper Soup	Campbell's	40.0	0.5	3.2	2.8	n/a
Mushroom & Wine Pasta 'n' Sauce, per packet, as served	Batchelors	546	21.0	106	9.2	10.7
Mushroom Carbonara Pasta Soup	Heinz	50.0	1.9	5.5	2.2	0.2
Mushroom Cup-A-Soup Special, per sachet	Batchelors	96.0	0.4	12.8	5.2	n/a
Mushroom Feasts, each	Birds Eye Country Club	100	2.0	12.0	5.0	0.9
Mushroom Ketchup	Burgess	27.0	0.4	5.5	0.1	Tr
Mushroom Pasta Sauce	Dolmio	36.0	0.9	8.2	Tr	n/a
Mushroom Pâté	Tartex	235	7.0	9.0	18.5	n/a
per tub	Vessen	120	2.9	5.8	9.4	0.1
Mushroom Ragu Sauce	Batchelors	64.0	2.0	8.7	2.3	n/a

All amounts given per 100g/100ml unless otherwise stated

Product	*Brand*	*Calories kcal*	*Protein (g)*	*Carbo-hydrate (g)*	*Fat (g)*	*Dietary Fibre (g)*
Mushroom Rice & Things Dry Mix, as sold	Crosse & Blackwell	370	9.6	75.7	3.1	2.2
Mushrooms						
common, raw		13.0	1.8	0.4	0.5	1.1
common, boiled		11.0	1.8	0.4	0.3	1.1
common, fried in oil		157	2.4	0.3	16.2	1.5
common, canned		12.0	2.1	Tr	0.4	1.3
Chinese, dried, raw		284	10.0	59.9	1.8	N
oyster, raw		8.0	1.6	Tr	0.2	N
shiitake, dried, raw		296	9.6	63.9	1.0	N
shiitake, cooked		55.0	1.6	12.3	0.2	N
straw, canned, drained		15.0	2.1	1.2	0.2	N
Mushroom Sauce Mix, as sold	Colman's	358	14.0	53.0	9.7	n/a
Mushroom Savoury Rice, per packet, as served	Batchelors	463	11.7	91.8	5.5	6.2
Mushroom Soup	Heinz Weight Watchers	24.0	1.0	3.5	0.6	0.1

dried, as sold	Knorr	353	10.7	64.2	5.9	n/a
per pack	Boots Shapers	40.00	n/a	n/a	1.0	n/a
Mushy Mint Peas	Batchelors	67.0	5.4	15.1	0.5	n/a
Mushy Peas, canned		81.0	5.8	13.8	0.7	1.8
	Batchelors	69.0	5.7	15.8	0.3	n/a
Mushy Peas Chip Shop Style	Batchelors	67.0	5.4	15.8	0.4	n/a
Mussels, boiled		87.0	17.2	Tr	2.0	nil
Mustard						
smooth		139	7.1	9.7	8.2	N
wholegrain		140	8.2	4.2	10.2	4.9
Mustard Dip, 28g/1oz	Kavli	98.0	n/a	n/a	n/a	n/a

All amounts given per 100g/100ml unless otherwise stated

N

Product	*Brand*	*Calories kcal*	*Protein (g)*	*Carbo-hydrate (g)*	*Fat (g)*	*Dietary Fibre (g)*
Naan Bread		336	8.9	50.1	12.5	1.9
Napoletana Pasta Sauce, chilled	Dolmio	49.0	1.3	7.0	1.8	n/a
Napoletana Pasta Sauce with Red Wine & Herbs (jar)	Dolmio	30.0	0.8	6.6	Tr	n/a
Napolitan Pasta Choice Dry Mix, as sold	Crosse & Blackwell	355	11.9	66.9	4.1	3.2
Natural Cod Steaks, each	Birds Eye Captain's Table	80.0	18.0	nil	0.5	nil
Natural Country Bran	Jordans	206	14.1	26.8	5.5	36.4
Natural Country Muesli	Jordans	350	10.2	64.1	5.9	7.4

Natural Harvest Processed Peas	Batchelors	77.0	5.8	17.2	0.6	n/a
Natural Soft Cheese, 28g/1oz	Primula	94.0	n/a	n/a	n/a	n/a
Natural Wheat Bran	Holland & Barrett	171	12.5	25.0	3.0	43.0
Natural Wheatgerm	Jordans	359	26.7	44.7	8.2	15.6
Natural Yogurt, Greek style	St Ivel	153	6.7	6.9	10.4	nil
Natural Yogurt, low fat	Holland & Barrett	65.0	5.7	8.3	1.0	nil
	St Ivel	64.0	5.6	6.5	1.2	nil
Neapolitan Dairy Ice Cream	Heinz Weight Watchers	135	3.3	16.9	5.6	0.3
Neapolitan Ice Cream	Fiesta	173	3.6	20.1	9.3	n/a
	Lyons Maid	87.0	1.8	11.0	4.0	n/a
Nectarine & Tangerine Yogurt	St Ivel Shape	43.0	4.6	5.9	0.1	0.2
Nectarine Bio Stirred Yogurt	Ski	112	5.8	16.7	2.9	nil

Product	*Brand*	*Calories kcal*	*Protein (g)*	*Carbo-hydrate (g)*	*Fat (g)*	*Dietary Fibre (g)*
Nectarines, flesh & skin		40.0	1.4	9.0	0.1	1.2
Neeps (England): *see Swede*						
Neeps (Scotland): *see Turnip*						
Nescafé Decaf	Nescafé	107	13.4	13.5	Tr	n/a
Nescafé Standard	Nescafé	94.0	12.6	11.0	Tr	nil
Nesquik (Nestlé): *see individual flavours*						
Nesquik Dessert	Chambourcy	190	5.3	21.2	9.5	Tr
New Orleans Chicken Simply Fix Dry Mix, as sold	Crosse & Blackwell	335	15.0	48.0	8.8	3.1
New Potatoes: *see Potatoes, new*						
Niblets	Green Giant	83.0	3.0	17.7	0.5	3.4
Niblets Lite	Green Giant	75.0	2.4	16.3	0.5	2.9
Nice 'n' Spicy Nik Naks, per pack	Golden Wonder	189	2.0	19.0	11.7	0.3

Nice 'n' Spicy Pot Noodle	Golden Wonder	407	12.0	61.7	12.4	n/a
Nice Biscuits	Jacob's	434	6.1	73.3	14.9	2.3
Nice Creams	Jacob's	487	5.7	67.8	21.9	2.0
95% Free Salad Cream Style Dressing	Kraft	75.0	0.4	6.8	4.8	1.4
No Bake Egg Custard Mix	Green's	109	3.5	13.5	4.5	n/a
Nobbly Bobbly, each	Lyons Maid	147	1.4	22.0	5.9	n/a
Non-dairy Ice Cream: *see Ice Cream*						
Noodles, egg, boiled		62.0	2.2	13.0	0.5	0.6
North Atlantic Peeled Prawns	Young's	61.0	15.1	nil	0.1	nil
No. 7 Cider	H P Bulmer	35.5	n/a	n/a	n/a	n/a
Nut & Chocolate Slices, each	Mr Kipling	150	3.6	13.6	9.4	n/a
Nut Crisp	Cadbury	525	8.5	53.9	30.6	n/a
Nut Feast	Kellogg's	390	11.0	68.0	8.0	7.0
Nut Meringue Gateau	McVitie's	407	3.0	32.4	29.5	Tr

All amounts given per 100g/100ml unless otherwise stated

Product	*Brand*	*Calories kcal*	*Protein (g)*	*Carbo-hydrate (g)*	*Fat (g)*	*Dietary Fibre (g)*
Nuts & Raisins, per pack	Golden Wonder	217	6.6	14.4	15.2	2.3
Nutty Crunchy Cereal	Holland & Barrett	361	10.5	60.0	12.0	12.0

O

Oat & Wheat Bran	Weetabix	334	11.7	60.2	5.2	16.9
Oat & Wheat Bran Hearts	Jordans	384	10.7	60.6	11.0	12.5
Oatbran	Jordans	340	17.0	55.0	9.0	15.0
	Mornflake	377	16.2	59.0	8.0	18.5
Oatbran & Apple Crunchy Bar	Jordans	452	8.2	59.6	20.1	6.2
Oatbran Ryvita, per slice	Ryvita	27.0	1.0	5.2	0.2	1.5
Oat Crispy Crunch	Mornflake	409	12.9	60.0	13.0	6.9
Oat Danish Bread	Heinz Weight Watchers	227	10.7	38.6	3.3	4.7
Oat Fingers, each	Paterson's	45.0	n/a	n/a	1.9	n/a

All amounts given per 100g/100ml unless otherwise stated

Product	Brand	Calories kcal	Protein (g)	Carbo-hydrate (g)	Fat (g)	Dietary Fibre (g)
Oat Flakes	Mornflake	385	11.8	68.0	7.3	7.2
Oat Krunchies	Quaker	394	8.8	76.0	5.5	5.1
Oatcakes		441	10.0	63.0	18.3	N
Oatmeal	Mornflake	385	11.8	68.0	7.3	7.2
Oatmeal Bread	Crofters Kitchen	234	8.1	41.6	3.9	3.7
Ocean Pie	Ross	121	7.0	9.8	6.2	0.4
Oily Mango Chutney	Burgess	241	0.3	58.6	Tr	0.8
OK Fruity Sauce	Colman's	95.0	0.9	24.0	0.2	n/a
Okra (gumbo, lady's fingers)						
boiled		28.0	2.5	2.7	0.9	3.6
stir-fried		269	4.3	4.4	26.1	6.3
canned, drained		21.0	1.4	2.5	0.7	2.6
Old Fashioned Jumbo Oats	Mornflake	385	11.8	68.0	7.3	7.2
Old Jamaica	Cadbury	465	5.8	57.0	23.7	n/a
Olive Oil		899	Tr	nil	99.9	nil

Olives, pitted, in brine		103	0.9	Tr	11.0	2.9
Olivio Reduced Fat Spread	Van Den Berghs	544	0.4	0.5	60.0	nil
Omelette, plain		191	10.9	Tr	16.4	nil
cheese		266	15.9	Tr	22.6	nil
Onion & Garlic Ragu Sauce	Batchelors	58.0	2.3	9.2	1.3	n/a
Onion Bhajia Mix	Sharwood	222	4.8	25.6	11.2	3.6
Onion Bhajis	Ross	151	5.7	25.8	3.9	2.5
Onion Crunchies	Ross	136	2.5	23.4	4.2	1.4
Onion Granules, as sold	Oxo	312	8.2	58.0	5.3	n/a
Onions						
raw		36.0	1.2	7.9	0.2	1.4
baked		103	3.5	22.3	0.6	3.9
boiled		17.0	0.6	3.7	0.1	0.7
fried in oil		164	2.3	14.1	11.2	3.1
dried, raw		313	10.2	68.6	1.7	12.1
pickled, drained		24.0	0.9	4.9	0.2	1.2
cocktail/silverskin, drained		15.0	0.6	3.1	0.1	N

All amounts given per 100g/100ml unless otherwise stated

Product	*Brand*	*Calories kcal*	*Protein (g)*	*Carbo-hydrate (g)*	*Fat (g)*	*Dietary Fibre (g)*
Onions & Garlic Ragu	Brooke Bond	80.0	1.8	12.6	2.8	n/a
Onion Sauce						
made with whole milk		99.0	2.8	8.3	6.5	0.4
made with semi-skimmed milk		86.0	2.9	8.4	5.0	0.4
Onion Sauce Mix, as sold	Colman's	316	8.3	68.0	1.0	n/a
	Knorr	348	8.1	65.7	5.9	n/a
Opal Fruits	Mars	411	0.3	85.3	7.6	n/a
Orangeade						
bottles	Corona	10.0	Tr	2.2	nil	n/a
cans	Corona	27.0	nil	6.6	nil	n/a
Orange Aero	Nestlé	520	7.7	58.0	28.6	n/a
Orange & Carob Crunchy Bar	Jordans	457	8.8	57.7	21.2	6.1
Orange & Lemon Crisp	Mornflake	466	9.9	70.3	16.2	6.3
Orange & Lemon Gateau	McVitie's	292	2.4	31.7	17.5	0.4
Orange & Lemon Torte	Heinz Weight Watchers	129	3.0	19.5	4.3	0.4

Orange & Lychee Yogurt	St Ivel Shape	43.0	4.6	5.9	0.1	0.1
Orange & Mango Special R, diluted	Robinsons	150	0.1	2.7	Tr	n/a
Orange & Peach C-Vit Ready to Drink	SmithKline Beecham	34.0	n/a	9.0	n/a	n/a
Orange & Pineapple Drink	Tango	46.0	Tr	11.1	Tr	n/a
low calorie	Tango	3.0	Tr	0.5	Tr	n/a
low calorie, diluted	Quosh	11.0	Tr	2.5	Tr	n/a
ready to drink	Quosh	18.0	Tr	4.2	Tr	n/a
sparkling	Tango	44.0	n/a	11.6	n/a	n/a
Orange & Pineapple Fruit Juice	Del Monte	42.0	0.5	10.8	Tr	n/a
Orange & Pineapple Special R, diluted	Robinsons	12.0	0.1	2.0	Tr	n/a
Orange & Pineapple Whole Fruit Drink, diluted	Robinsons	48.0	0.1	11.0	Tr	n/a
Orange & Raspberry Drink, per 250ml pack	Boots Shapers	111	n/a	n/a	Tr	n/a

All amounts given per 100g/100ml unless otherwise stated

Product	*Brand*	*Calories kcal*	*Protein (g)*	*Carbo-hydrate (g)*	*Fat (g)*	*Dietary Fibre (g)*
Orange & Walnut Crunchy	Mornflake	418	10.6	64.9	12.9	7.0
Orange Apple Passionfruit Juice	Del Monte	42.0	0.5	11.2	0.1	n/a
Orange Bar, each	Boots Shapers	96.0	n/a	n/a	3.8	n/a
Orange Barley Water, diluted	Robinsons	9.0	0.1	1.1	Tr	n/a
Orange 'C'	Libby	37.0	0.1	9.1	Tr	0.1
no added sugar	Libby	12.0	0.2	1.9	Tr	Tr
Orange Club Biscuits	Jacob's	511	5.8	61.5	26.8	1.2
Orange Cream	Cadbury	430	2.7	69.3	14.7	n/a
Orange Cream Biscuits	Cadbury	508	5.4	65.7	26.6	n/a
Orange Crush, per pack	Boots Shapers	22.0	n/a	n/a	Tr	n/a
Orange C-Vit	SmithKline Beecham	144	n/a	38.4	n/a	n/a
ready to drink	SmithKline Beecham	38.0	n/a	10.1	n/a	n/a

Orange Drink	Citrus Spring	41.0	Tr	9.9	Tr	n/a
	Jusoda	31.0	n/a	7.6	Tr	Tr
	Tango	48.0	Tr	11.6	Tr	n/a
undiluted		107	Tr	28.5	nil	nil
ready to drink	Quosh	19.6	Tr	4.4	Tr	n/a
per 250ml pack	Boots Shapers	113	n/a	n/a	Tr	n/a
low calorie, diluted	Quosh	1.0	Tr	0.1	Tr	n/a
low calorie, ready to drink	Quosh	5.0	Tr	4.4	nil	n/a
sparkling	St Clements	47.0	n/a	11.1	Tr	Tr
	Tango	46.0	n/a	12.3	n/a	n/a
Orange Flavour Jelly Crystals	Dietade	7.0	1.5	0.1	nil	nil
Orange Fruit Burst	Del Monte	38.0	0.2	9.8	Tr	n/a
Orange Fruit Juice	Del Monte	39.0	0.6	9.7	Tr	n/a
Orange Glucose Energy Tablets	Lucozade Sport	339	Tr	90.4	n/a	n/a
Orange Jelly, ready to eat	Rowntree	78.0	Tr	19.6	Tr	0.6
Orange Juice	Britvic 55	49.0	0.3	11.3	Tr	n/a
	Cawston Vale	43.0	0.6	10.5	Tr	n/a
ready to drink	Robinsons	41.0	Tr	98	Tr	n/a

All amounts given per 100g/100ml unless otherwise stated

Product	*Brand*	*Calories kcal*	*Protein (g)*	*Carbo-hydrate (g)*	*Fat (g)*	*Dietary Fibre (g)*
Orange Juice, unsweetened		36.0	0.5	8.8	0.1	0.1
Orange Maid, each	Lyons Maid	78.0	0.3	19.1	nil	n/a
Orange Marmalade, reduced sugar	Heinz Weight Watchers	127	0.2	31.4	nil	0.2
Orange Matchmakers	Nestlé	476	5.1	68.5	20.2	n/a
Orange Mr Men, each	Lyons Maid	28.0	nil	7.0	nil	n/a
Orange Peach Apricot Juice	Del Monte	39.0	0.6	9.7	Tr	n/a
Orange Puff	Jacob's	486	5.9	66.1	22.0	1.6
Oranges, flesh only		37.0	1.1	8.5	0.1	1.7
Orange Sorbet Fromage Frais	St Ivel Shape	51.0	6.2	6.3	0.1	0.1
Orange Special R, diluted	Robinsons	31.0	Tr	n/a	n/a	n/a
ready to drink	Robinsons	4.7	0.1	0.8	Tr	n/a
Orange Squash, low calorie	Dietade	12.0	nil	2.4	Tr	n/a
Orange Squash, undiluted	St Clements	120	0.7	31.8	0.1	n/a

Orange Whole Fruit Drink, diluted	Robinsons	48.0	0.1	11.0	Tr	n/a
Orange Yogurt	Ski	88.0	5.0	16.4	0.7	nil
Orange YoYo	McVitie's	523	4.7	63.8	27.6	1.0
Orbit Chewing Gum						
Fruit	Wrigley	180	nil	52.0	nil	nil
Peppermint	Wrigley	190	nil	63.0	nil	nil
Spearmint	Wrigley	195	nil	64.0	nil	nil
Orchards Pie	McVitie's	272	3.8	38.4	12.0	1.1
Oregano, fresh		66.0	2.2	9.7	2.0	N
dried, ground		306	11.0	49.5	10.3	N
Organio Cats	Mornflake	385	11.8	68.0	7.3	7.2
Oriental Beef Stir Fry Mix, as sold	Crosse & Blackwell	370	7.7	65.3	8.8	1.5
Oriental Chicken Cup Noodle	Golden Wonder	427	8.5	61.9	16.1	n/a
Oriental Chicken Microchef Meal	Batchelors	83.0	6.0	12.9	1.2	n/a

Product	*Brand*	*Calories kcal*	*Protein (g)*	*Carbo-hydrate (g)*	*Fat (g)*	*Dietary Fibre (g)*
Oriental Chicken Stir Fry Mix, as sold	Crosse & Blackwell	385	7.1	61.8	12.3	1.8
Oriental Mix	Ross	43.0	2.0	9.4	0.3	1.3
Oriental Sweet & Sour Chicken Tonight Sauce	Batchelors	97.0	0.4	23.6	0.1	n/a
Oriental Sweet & Sour Cooking Sauce	Heinz Weight Watchers	43.0	0.9	9.5	0.2	0.7
Original Barbecue American Sauce	Heinz	94.0	1.0	22.2	0.1	0.5
Original Barbecue Sauce	Lea & Perrins	140	1.1	32.1	0.8	n/a
Original Beef Granules, as sold	Oxo	294	12.0	54.5	4.7	n/a
Original Cider	H P Bulmer	36.8	n/a	n/a	n/a	n/a
Original Crunchy Cereal with Raisins & Rippled Almond	Jordans	387	9.4	62.6	11.0	9.5
Original Crunchy Cereal with						

Tropical Fruits	Jordans	422	8.6	62.1	15.5	8.0
Original French Dressing	Kraft	496	Tr	5.0	54.0	nil
Original Fruit Drink	Rowntree	49.0	Tr	12.0	Tr	nil
Original Glucose Energy Tablets	Lucozade Sport	339	nil	90.4	n/a	n/a
Original Italian Garlic Dressing	Kraft	426	Tr	7.0	43.0	0.1
Original Mixed Vegetables, 1oz/28g	Birds Eye Country Club	15.0	1.0	2.5	0.1	0.9
Original Oatcakes, each	Vessen	115	2.9	15.3	4.5	1.6
Original Pasta Sauce	Dolmio	37.0	0.9	8.4	Tr	n/a
Lite	Dolmio	24.0	0.8	5.2	Tr	n/a
with Mushrooms	Dolmio	36.0	0.9	7.9	Tr	n/a
with Spicy Peppers	Dolmio	36.0	0.9	8.2	Tr	n/a
Original Ryvita, per slice	Ryvita	25.0	0.7	5.6	0.2	1.3
Outline Very Low Fat Spread	Van Den Berghs	222	3.5	1.5	22.5	nil

All amounts given per 100g/100ml unless otherwise stated

Product	*Brand*	*Calories kcal*	*Protein (g)*	*Carbo-hydrate (g)*	*Fat (g)*	*Dietary Fibre (g)*
Ovaltine, powder		358	9.0	79.4	2.7	N
made up with whole milk		97.0	3.8	12.9	3.8	Tr
made up with semi-skimmed milk		79.0	3.9	13.0	1.7	Tr
Oven Chips	Ross	131	2.4	20.6	5.1	1.6
Oven Crispy Cod Fish Fingers, each	Birds Eye Captain's Table	85.0	3.5	4.0	4.0	0.1
Oven Crispy Cod Steaks, each	Birds Eye Captain's Table	235	12.0	13.0	15.0	0.2
Oven Crispy Haddock Steaks, each	Birds Eye Captain's Table	235	12.0	13.0	15.0	0.2
Oven Crunchies	Ross	188	2.7	24.5	8.7	1.9
Oxo Beef Drink, as served	Brooke Bond	3.9	0.7	0.2	nil	n/a
Oxo Cubes, as sold	Brooke Bond	272	17.7	41.1	4.8	n/a
Oxtail, stewed		243	30.5	nil	13.4	nil
Oxtail Cup-A-Soup, per sachet	Batchelors	77.0	1.2	13.8	2.3	n/a

Oxtail Quick Soup	Knorr	358	10.7	53.3	11.3	n/a
Oxtail Soup, dried, as served		27.0	1.4	3.9	0.8	N
	Knorr	327	11.5	57.5	5.7	n/a
Oxtail Soup, dried, as sold		356	17.6	51.0	10.5	N
canned	Campbell's	38.0	1.5	5.2	1.3	n/a
	Crosse & Blackwell	34.0	2.0	5.1	0.6	0.2
	Heinz	55.0	1.5	5.3	1.2	0.2

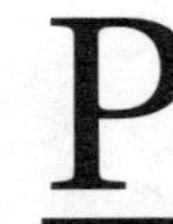

Product	*Brand*	*Calories kcal*	*Protein (g)*	*Carbo-hydrate (g)*	*Fat (g)*	*Dietary Fibre (g)*
Pacific Salmon Slices	Young's	182	18.4	nil	12.0	nil
Paella	Vesta	123	4.4	20.1	3.3	n/a
per single serving	Vesta	294	11.1	54.6	3.4	n/a
Fast Cook	Ross	93.0	5.6	15.6	1.4	0.9
Paglia e Fieno, as sold	Dolmio	125	4.6	25.6	1.2	n/a
Pale Ale, bottled		32.0	0.3	2.0	Tr	nil
Paleskin Peanuts	Holland & Barrett	564	25.6	12.5	46.1	7.3
Palm Oil		899	Tr	nil	99.9	nil
Pancake Mix	Whitworths	322	13.4	65.9	2.5	2.3

Food	Brand					
Pancake Roll		217	6.6	20.9	12.5	N
Pancakes						
savoury, made with whole milk		273	6.3	24.0	17.5	0.8
sweet, made with whole milk		301	5.9	35.0	16.2	0.8
Papaya, unripe, raw		27.0	0.9	5.5	0.1	1.5
Papaya/Pineapple in Light Syrup	Del Monte	64.0	0.6	16.3	Tr	n/a
Parmesan Cheese		452	39.4	Tr	32.7	nil
	Napolina	480	46.0	Tr	37.0	n/a
Parmesan Style Ragu	Brooke Bond	90.0	2.9	12.1	2.6	n/a
Parmesan with Garlic Pasta 'n' Sauce, per packet, as served	Batchelors	512	22.9	93.1	9.4	8.6
Parsley Pour Over Sauce	Knorr	73.0	2.2	8.1	3.8	Tr
Parsley Sauce Mix, as sold	Colman's	320	10.0	66.0	1.7	n/a
	Knorr	342	5.3	58.8	9.5	n/a
Parsnip, boiled		66.0	1.6	12.9	1.2	4.7
Partridge, roast, meat only		212	36.7	nil	7.2	nil

All amounts given per 100g/100ml unless otherwise stated

Product	*Brand*	*Calories kcal*	*Protein (g)*	*Carbo-hydrate (g)*	*Fat (g)*	*Dietary Fibre (g)*
Party Parade, each	Nestlé	153	2.9	15.7	7.2	n/a
Party Size Sausage Rolls	Kraft	320	6.6	24.7	22.3	n/a
Passanda Classic Curry Sauce	Homepride	103	2.5	12.8	4.5	n/a
Passionfruit, flesh & pips only		36.0	2.6	5.8	0.4	3.3
Passionfruit Country Crisp	Jordans	435	3.7	32.3	8.2	4.0
Passionfruit Melba Yogurt	St Ivel Shape	41.0	4.6	5.5	0.1	0.7
Pasta, cooked, all shapes						
egg	Buitoni	132	5.2	24.4	1.5	1.3
standard	Buitoni	129	4.8	25.9	0.7	1.2
Pasta Bolognese	Heinz Weight Watchers	85.0	5.0	11.9	2.0	0.8
Pasta Bolognese Microchef Meal	Batchelors	114	5.9	13.4	4.5	n/a
Pasta Choice (Crosse & Blackwell): ***see individual flavours***						
Pasta Pipes with Tuna & Bacon	Heinz	72.0	4.1	10.4	1.5	0.9

Pasta Salad	Heinz	194	2.3	21.4	11.0	0.7
Pasta Sauce, tomato based		47.0	2.0	6.9	1.5	N
Pasta Shells in Cheese & Tomato Sauce	Heinz	107	2.8	14.0	4.4	0.7
Pasta Shells with Vegetables & Prawns	Heinz Weight Watchers	76.0	3.7	10.9	2.1	0.7
Pasta Supreme Casserole Mix, as sold	Colman's	410	11.0	55.0	16.0	n/a
Pasta Tubes in Cheese Sauce with Bacon Italiana	Heinz Weight Watchers	74.0	4.2	7.8	2.8	0.2
Pasties: *see individual flavours*						
Pastilles		253	5.2	61.9	nil	nil
Pastries: *see individual flavours*						
Pastry						
flaky, cooked		560	5.6	45.9	40.6	1.4
shortcrust, cooked		521	6.6	54.2	32.3	2.2
wholemeal, cooked		499	8.9	44.6	32.9	6.3

All amounts given per 100g/100ml unless otherwise stated

Product	Brand	Calories kcal	Protein (g)	Carbo-hydrate (g)	Fat (g)	Dietary Fibre (g)
Pâté: ***see individual flavours***						
Patent Cornflour	Brown & Polson	343	0.6	83.6	0.7	n/a
Pavlova: ***see individual flavours***						
Paw-paw, raw		36.0	0.5	8.8	0.1	2.2
canned in juice		65.0	0.2	17.0	Tr	0.7
Pea & Ham Soup	Baxters	75.0	3.1	9.7	2.9	1.5
	Heinz Wholesoup	54.0	3.0	8.0	1.1	0.9
Peach & Apricot Torte	Heinz Weight Watchers	138	3.2	20.3	4.9	0.4
Peach & Goldenberry Yogurt	St Ivel Shape	42.0	4.6	5.7	0.1	0.1
Peach & Raspberry Layer Pies, each	Mr Kipling	203	2.1	33.7	2.1	n/a
Peach & Vanilla Yogurt, per pack	Boots Shapers	61.0	n/a	n/a	0.1	n/a

Food	Brand					
Peach Chutney	Sharwood	163	0.7	39.8	0.1	2.1
Peaches						
raw		33.0	1.0	7.6	0.1	1.5
canned in natural juice		39.0	0.6	9.7	Tr	0.8
canned in syrup		55.0	0.5	14.0	Tr	0.9
Peach Fromage Frais	Ski	124	6.2	14.2	4.8	n/a
Peach Halves in Natural Juice	Libby	51.0	0.4	12.4	Tr	0.3
in Syrup	Libby	82.0	0.5	20.0	Tr	0.3
Peach Melba Ice Cream	Lyons Maid	94.0	1.7	13.2	3.8	n/a
Peach Melba Long Life Yogurt	St Ivel Prize	69.0	3.4	13.8	0.1	0.5
Peach Melba Split Sundae, per pack	Boots Shapers	82.0	n/a	n/a	4.2	n/a
Peach Melba Yogurt	St Ivel Shape	41.0	4.5	5.5	0.1	0.2
Peach Slices in Natural Juice	Libby	52.0	0.4	12.4	0.1	0.3
in Syrup	Libby	82.0	0.4	20.0	Tr	0.3
Peach Spring, per pack	Boots Shapers	3.0	n/a	n/a	Tr	n/a

All amounts given per 100g/100ml unless otherwise stated

Product	Brand	Calories kcal	Protein (g)	Carbo-hydrate (g)	Fat (g)	Dietary Fibre (g)
Peach Trifle	St Ivel	152	1.5	24.7	5.4	0.3
Peach Yogurt	Ski	94.0	5.1	17.0	1.1	nil
Peanut Bar, each	Boots Shapers	98.0	n/a	n/a	3.8	n/a
Peanut Butter, Smooth		623	22.6	13.1	53.7	5.4
Peanut Harvest Crunch Bar, each	Quaker	109	2.6	13.2	4.8	0.9
Peanut M & Ms	Mars	514	10.2	57.3	27.1	n/a
Peanut Oil		899	Tr	nil	99.9	nil
Peanuts						
plain, kernel only		564	25.6	12.5	46.1	6.2
dry roasted		589	25.5	10.3	49.8	6.4
roasted & salted		602	24.5	7.1	53.0	6.0
Peanuts & Raisins	Holland & Barrett	465	17.6	31.8	30.6	6.9
Peanut Yorkie	Nestlé	542	11.6	48.4	33.6	n/a

Pear & Apple Juice	Copella	39.0	n/a	10.1	nil	nil
Pear Drops	Cravens	386	Tr	96.4	nil	nil
each	Trebor Bassett	15.9	nil	3.9	nil	nil
Pear Halves in Syrup	Libby	77.0	0.1	19.2	Tr	0.6
in Natural Juice	Libby	54.0	0.1	13.3	Tr	0.5
Pearl Barley	Whitworths	360	7.9	83.6	1.7	7.3
Pears						
raw, average		40.0	0.3	10.0	0.1	2.2
canned in natural juice		33.0	0.3	8.5	Tr	1.4
canned in syrup		50.0	0.2	13.2	Tr	1.1
Peas						
boiled		79.0	6.7	10.0	1.6	4.5
dried, boiled		109	6.9	19.9	0.8	5.5
frozen, boiled		69.0	6.0	9.7	0.9	5.1
canned		80.0	5.3	13.5	0.9	5.1
Peas & Baby Carrots, 1oz/28g	Birds Eye Country Club	11.0	1.0	1.5	0.1	1.1
Pea with Ham Quick Soup	Knorr	364	15.4	47.4	12.5	n/a

All amounts given per 100g/100ml unless otherwise stated

Product	*Brand*	*Calories kcal*	*Protein (g)*	*Carbo-hydrate (g)*	*Fat (g)*	*Dietary Fibre (g)*
Pecan Nuts		689	9.2	5.8	70.1	4.7
Peeled Plum Tomatoes	Napolina	12.0	1.1	2.0	Tr	n/a
Peking Barbecue Spare Ribs	Knorr	85.0	0.8	18.9	1.2	0.5
Penguin Biscuits	McVitie's	448	5.3	70.0	16.5	1.1
Peppercorn Pâté, per pack	Boots Shapers	140	n/a	n/a	8.3	n/a
Peppered Grillsteak	Ross	311	15.3	1.7	27.0	nil
Peppermint Chewing Gum (Wrigley): ***see Chewing Gum***						
Peppermint Cordial, diluted	Britvic	19.0	nil	4.8	Tr	n/a
Peppermint Cream	Cadbury	430	2.7	69.7	14.7	n/a
Peppermints		392	0.5	102.2	0.7	nil
Pepperoni & Sausage Pizza	San Marco	226	10.9	24.8	9.9	1.3
Pepperoni Deep Crust Pizza	McCain	227	10.3	30.4	7.2	n/a
Pepperoni Deep Pan Pizza	McCain	227	10.3	30.4	7.2	n/a
Pepperoni French Bread	Heinz Weight					

Pizza	Watchers	157	11.0	15.4	5.7	2.6
Pepperoni, Ham & Mushroom Single Serve Pizza	McCain	219	10.9	25.8	7.3	n/a
Pepperoni, Ham & Spicy Beef Micro Pizza	McCain	206	12.7	29.7	4.8	n/a
Pepperoni Pizza Rolla	McCain	219	10.9	24.0	9.6	n/a
Pepperoni Pizza Slice	McCain	214	10.1	24.6	8.6	n/a
Pepper Pâté	Tartex	242	7.0	13.0	18.5	n/a
per tub	Vessen	97.0	2.7	4.1	7.8	0.2
Peppers						
green, raw		15.0	0.8	2.6	0.3	1.6
green, boiled		18.0	1.0	2.6	0.5	1.8
red, raw		32.0	1.0	6.4	0.4	1.6
red, boiled		34.0	1.1	7.0	0.4	1.7
yellow, raw		26.0	1.2	5.3	0.2	1.7
Peppers Mustard	Colman's	194	7.0	18.0	9.6	n/a
Pepsi Cola	Pepsi	44.0	nil	11.1	nil	n/a
Diet Pepsi	Pepsi	0.25	0.1	0.1	nil	n/a

All amounts given per 100g/100ml unless otherwise stated

Product	*Brand*	*Calories kcal*	*Protein (g)*	*Carbo-hydrate (g)*	*Fat (g)*	*Dietary Fibre (g)*
Perkins	Tunnock's	429	7.4	77.4	12.0	n/a
Petits Pois, frozen, boiled		49.0	5.0	5.5	0.9	4.5
canned		45.0	5.2	4.9	0.6	4.3
Petit Pois	Ross	51.0	4.2	10.4	1.2	4.6
Pheasant, roast, meat only		213	32.2	nil	9.3	nil
Philadelphia Full Fat Soft Cheese	Kraft	310	8.0	3.0	30.0	0.3
Philadelphia Light Medium Fat Soft Cheese	Kraft	185	9.0	3.5	15.0	0.4
with Pineapple	Kraft	185	7.6	12.6	11.5	0.1
with Salmon	Kraft	187	9.0	3.5	15.0	0.6
Piccalilli	Heinz Ploughman's	89.0	1.2	20.0	0.3	0.5
Pickle, sweet		134	0.6	34.4	0.3	1.2
Pickle with Worcestershire Sauce	Lea & Perrins	150	0.9	33.6	1.3	n/a

Pickled Beetroot: ***see Beetroot***						
Pickled Gherkin: ***see Gherkins***						
Pickled Onion Crisps, per pack	Golden Wonder	152	2.0	12.2	10.6	1.3
Pickled Onion Nik Naks, per pack	Golden Wonder	199	1.7	18.2	13.3	0.3
Pickled Onions: ***see Onions***						
Pickled Onion Snakebites, per pack	Golden Wonder	95.0	1.0	11.2	5.1	0.2
Picnic	Cadbury	475	7.9	58.9	23.4	n/a
Pigeon, roast, meat only		230	27.8	nil	13.2	nil
Pikelets	Sunblest	182	5.9	37.5	0.9	1.4
Pilau Delicately Flavoured Rice, per packet, as served	Batchelors	849	18.2	183	8.1	11.5
Pilau Rice	Sharwood	353	8.6	76.8	1.2	1.8
frozen	Uncle Ben's	148	3.4	30.5	1.4	n/a

All amounts given per 100g/100ml unless otherwise stated

Product	Brand	Calories kcal	Protein (g)	Carbo-hydrate (g)	Fat (g)	Dietary Fibre (g)
Pilchards, canned in tomato sauce		126	18.8	0.7	5.4	Tr
Pina Colada, per pack	Boots Shapers	33.0	n/a	n/a	nil	n/a
Pinacolada Fromage Frais	St Ivel Shape	55.0	6.2	6.8	0.3	0.2
Pineapple						
raw		41.0	0.4	10.1	0.2	1.2
canned in natural juice		47.0	0.3	12.2	Tr	0.5
canned in syrup		64.0	0.5	16.5	Tr	0.7
Pineapple & Cream Mivi, each	Lyons Maid	85.0	1.0	13.8	2.8	n/a
Pineapple & Ginger Stir Fry Sauce	Homepride	91.0	0.3	22.9	0.1	n/a
Pineapple & Grapefruit Drink	Tango	44.0	Tr	11.8	Tr	n/a
Pineapple & Pepper Relish	Colman's	214	0.4	52.0	Tr	n/a
Pineapple & Ruby Grapefruit						

Drink, per pack	Boots Shapers	54.0	n/a	n/a	Tr	n/a
Pineapple 'C'	Libby	44.0	0.1	10.9	Tr	Tr
Pineapple Chunks, each	Trebor Bassett	18.2	nil	4.5	nil	nil
Pineapple Chunks in Juice	Del Monte	63.0	0.4	16.0	0.2	n/a
Pineapple Cottage Cheese	St Ivel Shape	72.0	8.7	9.2	0.1	Tr
Pineapple Crusha	Burgess	117	Tr	29.3	nil	nil
Pineapple Fruit Juice	Del Monte	46.0	0.3	11.9	Tr	n/a
Pineapple Juice	Britvic 55	51.0	0.1	13.6	Tr	n/a
Pineapple Juice, unsweetened		41.0	0.3	10.5	0.1	Tr
Pineapple Juice Carton	Robinsons	38.0	Tr	9.2	Tr	n/a
Pineapple Rings						
in natural juice	Libby	50.0	n/a	n/a	Tr	n/a
in syrup	Libby	80.0	0.4	19.6	Tr	0.4
Pineapple Yogurt	Ski	96.0	5.0	17.4	1.1	nil
Pine Nuts		688	14.0	4.0	68.6	1.9

All amounts given per 100g/100ml unless otherwise stated

Product	Brand	Calories kcal	Protein (g)	Carbo-hydrate (g)	Fat (g)	Dietary Fibre (g)
Pinto Beans, dried, boiled		137	8.9	23.9	0.7	N
refried		107	6.2	15.3	1.1	N
Pistachio Nuts, weighed with shells		331	9.9	4.6	30.5	3.3
Pitta Bread, white		265	9.2	57.9	1.2	2.2
Pizza: *see flavours*						
Pizza Bases	Napolina	280	8.5	55.8	4.1	n/a
Pizza Style Club Sandwiches, per pack	Boots Shapers	186	n/a	n/a	n/a	n/a
Pizza Toppings Tomato, Cheese, Onion & Herbs	Napolina	79.0	2.1	10.1	3.4	n/a
Pizza Topping, Tomato, Herbs & Spices	Napolina	64.0	1.3	11.3	1.8	n/a
PK Chewing Gum, all flavours	Wrigley	330	nil	82.0	nil	nil
Plaice, steamed		93.0	18.9	nil	1.9	nil
in batter, fried in oil		279	15.8	14.4	18.0	N
in crumbs, fried, fillets		228	18.0	8.6	13.7	N

Plain Chocolate		525	4.7	64.8	29.2	N
Plain Wholewheat Flapjack	Holland & Barrett	490	5.3	54.9	27.7	4.6
Ploughman's Pickles, Sauces, etc. (Heinz): ***see individual flavours***						
Plum Chinese Spare Rib Sauce	Sharwood	241	0.5	59.4	0.2	0.6
Plums, average, raw		36.0	0.6	8.8	0.1	1.6
canned in syrup		59.0	0.3	15.5	Tr	0.8
Poached Salmon with Chinese Leaf Sandwiches, per pack	Boots Shapers	198	n/a	n/a	n/a	n/a
Polo Fruits	Nestlé	384	nil	96.0	nil	n/a
Polo Mints	Nestlé	404	1.1	97.3	1.1	n/a
Polony		281	9.4	14.2	21.1	N
Pontefract Cakes, each	Trebor Bassett	7.6	nil	1.8	nil	nil
Popcorn, candied		480	2.1	77.6	20.0	N
plain		592	6.2	48.6	42.8	N

Product	*Brand*	*Calories kcal*	*Protein (g)*	*Carbo-hydrate (g)*	*Fat (g)*	*Dietary Fibre (g)*
Popcorn Prawns	Lyons Seafoods	280	9.1	18.9	19.4	n/a
Poppadums, fried in veg. oil		369	17.5	39.1	16.9	N
	Sharwood	281	20.4	45.6	1.9	10.3
Poppets Peanut Assortment	G. Payne & Co	536	14.0	43.0	35.0	n/a
Poppets Peanuts	G. Payne & Co	562	17.0	36.0	39.0	n/a
Poppets Peanuts & Raisins	G. Payne & Co	482	11.0	50.0	27.0	n/a
Poppets Raisins	G. Payne & Co	403	5.1	64.0	14.0	n/a
Poppets White Raisins	G. Payne & Co	442	6.3	62.0	19.0	n/a
Pork, belly rashers						
lean & fat, grilled		398	21.1	nil	34.8	nil
Pork, chops						
loin, lean only, grilled		226	32.3	nil	10.7	nil
Pork, leg						
lean & fat, roast		286	26.9	nil	19.8	nil
lean only, roast		185	30.7	nil	6.9	nil

Pork, trotters & tails salted, boiled		280	19.8	nil	22.3	nil
Pork Casserole Mix, as sold	Colman's	214	6.6	64.0	1.4	n/a
Pork Pie, individual		376	9.8	24.9	27.0	0.9
Pork Sausages: *see Sausages*						
Pork Stock Cubes	Knorr	354	9.3	27.3	23.1	n/a
Porridge, made with water		49.0	1.5	9.0	1.0	0.8
made with whole milk		116	4.8	13.7	5.1	0.8
Porridge Oats	Whitworths	401	12.4	72.8	8.7	7.0
Port		157	0.1	12.0	nil	nil
Postman Pat Choc Candy, each	Trebor Bassett	35.0	0.3	4.0	1.9	nil
Potato & Ham Gratin	Findus Dinner Supreme	118	6.4	6.5	7.6	1.9
Potato & Leek Soup	Baxters	36.0	0.6	7.1	0.7	0.8
	Heinz Farmhouse	34.0	0.7	6.4	0.6	0.5

All amounts given per 100g/100ml unless otherwise stated

Product	Brand	Calories kcal	Protein (g)	Carbo-hydrate (g)	Fat (g)	Dietary Fibre (g)
Potato Cakes	Sunblest	255	4.6	32.7	11.7	1.9
Potato Crisps		546	5.6	49.3	37.6	4.9
low fat		483	6.6	63.0	21.5	6.3
Potato Croquettes, fried in oil		214	3.7	21.6	13.1	1.3
Potatoes, new						
boiled		75.0	1.5	17.8	0.3	1.1
boiled in skins		66.0	1.4	15.4	0.3	1.5
canned		63.0	1.5	15.1	0.1	0.8
Potatoes, old						
baked, flesh & skin		136	3.9	31.7	0.2	2.7
baked, flesh only		77.0	2.2	18.0	0.1	1.4
boiled		72.0	1.8	17.0	0.1	1.2
mashed with margarine & milk		104	1.8	15.5	4.3	1.1
roast in oil/lard		149	2.9	25.9	4.5	1.8
Potato Hoops		523	3.9	58.5	32.0	2.6
Potato Pancakes	Ross	239	3.2	18.8	17.4	1.3

Potato Pancakes with Onion	Ross	228	2.9	22.0	15.2	2.2
Potato Powder: ***see Instant Potato Powder***						
Potato Salad	Heinz	176	1.7	15.2	10.5	0.8
Potato Waffles, frozen, cooked		200	3.2	30.3	8.2	2.3
	Ross	225	2.3	22.0	12.3	2.0
each	Birds Eye Country Club	110	1.5	15.0	5.0	1.1
Potted Shrimps	Young's	358	16.5	nil	32.4	nil
Pouring Syrup (Lyle's): ***see individual flavours***						
Prawn & Cucumber Bap, each	Boots Shapers	176	n/a	n/a	n/a	n/a
Prawn & Cucumber/Turkey & Chinese Leaf/Smoked Ham & Salad Triple Pack Sandwiches, per pack	Boots Shapers	291	n/a	n/a	n/a	n/a
Prawn & Egg Sandwiches, per pack	Boots Shapers	255	n/a	n/a	n/a	n/a

All amounts given per 100g/100ml unless otherwise stated

Product	*Brand*	*Calories kcal*	*Protein (g)*	*Carbo-hydrate (g)*	*Fat (g)*	*Dietary Fibre (g)*
Prawn, Apple & Celery/Tuna Mayonnaise & Cucumber/ Seafood Cocktail Triple Sandwiches, per pack	Boots Shapers	292	n/a	n/a	n/a	n/a
Prawn, Apple & Celery with Soft Cheese Sandwiches, per pack	Boots Shapers	178	n/a	n/a	n/a	n/a
Prawn Cocktail	Lyons Seafoods	429	5.7	4.5	42.9	n/a
Prawn Cocktail Crisps, per bag	Golden Wonder	151	2.0	12.1	10.5	1.3
Prawn Cocktail Sauce	Burgess	338	2.5	16.2	28.5	0.5
Prawn Crackers	Sharwood	296	1.0	69.4	0.5	1.7
Prawn Curry	Findus Dinner Supreme	110	4.3	18.0	2.3	0.8
	Ross	117	5.0	21.5	1.4	0.4
with rice	Findus Lean Cuisine	92.0	5.1	12.3	2.5	1.1

per pack	Birds Eye Menu Master	405	14.0	63.0	11.0	4.0
Prawn Jal Frezzi Platter, per meal	Birds Eye Healthy Options	365	17.0	54.0	9.0	2.8
Prawn Kievs	Lyons Seafoods	224	9.1	16.0	13.8	n/a
Prawns, boiled		107	22.6	nil	1.8	nil
	Lyons Seafoods	61.0	13.5	nil	0.6	n/a
Premier Protein Biscuit Cakes	Itona	500	15.0	50.0	26.0	n/a
Premier Protein Chocolate Biscuit Cakes	Itona	530	13.1	47.0	32.2	n/a
Premium Choice Broccoli Spears	Ross	24.0	2.9	4.1	0.7	2.6
Premium Choice Brussels Sprouts	Ross	35.0	4.1	6.6	0.5	3.2
Premium Lemonade	R Whites	28.0	Tr	6.8	Tr	n/a
low calorie	R Whites	1.0	Tr	Tr	Tr	n/a

All amounts given per 100g/100ml unless otherwise stated

Product	*Brand*	*Calories kcal*	*Protein (g)*	*Carbo-hydrate (g)*	*Fat (g)*	*Dietary Fibre (g)*
Premium Scampi Tails	Lyons Seafoods	230	8.4	26.0	10.9	n/a
Preserving Sugar	Tate & Lyle	400	nil	99.9	nil	nil
Prime Cod Fish Fingers, each	Birds Eye Captain's Table	45.0	3.0	2.0	4.0	n/a
	Steakhouse	225	19.0	1.5	16.0	0.2
Prizeburgers, each	Birds Eye Steakhouse	212	20.0	3.5	14.0	0.8
Prizegrill Grillsteaks, each	Birds Eye					
Prizegrill Platter, per pack	Birds Eye Menu Master	540	26.0	33.0	34.0	4.0
Processed Cheese, plain		330	20.8	0.9	27.0	nil
Processed Cheese Slices, reduced fat	Heinz Weight Watchers	197	26.5	0.2	10.0	nil
Processed Peas, canned		99.0	6.9	17.5	0.7	4.8
Profiteroles	McVitie's	358	6.2	18.5	29.2	0.4

Promise 97% Fat Free Spread	Van Den Berghs	75.0	2.4	9.0	3.0	4.5
Provençal Pâté, per pack	Boots Shapers	131	n/a	n/a	7.5	n/a
Provençale Pour Over Sauce	Baxters	67.0	1.6	8.6	2.9	0.5
Prunes						
canned in juice		79.0	0.7	19.7	0.2	2.4
canned in syrup		90.0	0.6	23.0	0.2	2.8
ready to eat		141	2.5	34.0	0.4	5.7
Puffed Wheat		321	14.2	67.3	1.3	5.6
Pumpkin, raw		13.0	0.7	2.2	0.2	1.0
boiled		13.0	0.6	2.1	0.3	1.1
Pumpkin Seeds	Holland & Barrett	579	29.0	8.0	47.0	8.0
Pure Unsweetened Orange Juice	Holland & Barrett	43.0	0.7	10.4	Tr	nil

All amounts given per 100g/100ml unless otherwise stated

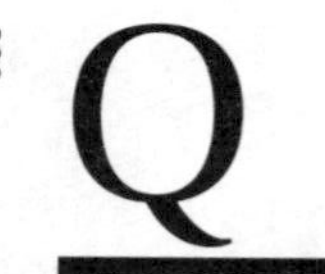

Product	Brand	Calories kcal	Protein (g)	Carbo-hydrate (g)	Fat (g)	Dietary Fibre (g)
Quaker Feast of Flakes	Quaker	381	8.0	76.0	5.0	4.4
Quaker Oat Bran	Quaker	347	13.0	54.5	8.2	10.3
Quaker Oat Bran Crispies	Quaker	370	12.2	68.8	4.6	9.0
Quaker Oats	Quaker	375	10.0	70.2	7.4	7.0
Quaker Puffed Wheat	Quaker	328	15.3	62.4	1.3	5.6
Quaker Wholegrain Feast	Quaker	385	9.7	65.0	9.5	7.8
Quality Street	Nestlé	451	3.9	68.5	17.9	n/a
Quarter Pounder, each	McDonald's	411	23.6	29.7	22.0	4.0
with cheese, each	McDonald's	501	29.2	33.7	27.7	5.6

Quenchers	Trebor Bassett	332	3.6	80.0	nil	nil
Quiche						
cheese & egg		314	12.5	17.3	22.2	0.6
cheese & egg, wholemeal		308	13.2	14.5	22.4	1.9
Quorn, myco-protein		86.0	11.8	2.0	3.5	4.8
Quosh Fruit Drinks: ***see individual flavours***						

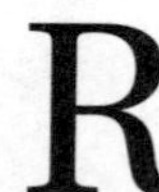

Product	Brand	Calories kcal	Protein (g)	Carbo-hydrate (g)	Fat (g)	Dietary Fibre (g)
Rabbit, stewed, meat only		179	27.3	nil	7.7	nil
Raddiccio, raw		14.0	1.4	1.7	0.2	1.8
Radish, red, raw		12.0	0.7	1.9	0.2	0.9
white/mooli, raw		15.0	0.8	2.9	0.1	N
Ragu Pasta Sauces: *see individual flavours*						
Rainbow Trout	Young's	89.0	13.8	nil	3.8	nil
Raisin & Biscuit Yorkie	Nestlé	481	6.3	60.5	23.8	n/a
Raisin & Hazelnut Frusli Bar	Jordans	431	6.5	62.7	17.1	4.0
Raisin & Lemon Pancakes	Sunblest	275	6.3	51.4	4.9	1.7

Raisin & Rum Cakes	Mr Kipling	92.0	0.7	10.5	4.7	n/a
Raisins		272	2.1	69.3	0.4	2.0
Raisins & Peanuts		435	15.3	37.5	26.0	4.4
Raisin Splitz	Kellogg's	320	9.0	69.0	1.5	8.0
Rambutans & Pineapple in Syrup	Libby	74.0	n/a	n/a	Tr	n/a
Rapeseed Oil		899	Tr	nil	99.9	nil
Raspberries, raw		7.0	0.9	0.8	0.1	2.5
stewed with sugar		48.0	0.9	11.5	0.1	1.2
stewed without sugar		7.0	0.9	0.7	0.1	1.3
canned in syrup		31.0	0.5	7.6	Tr	0.8
Raspberry & Apple Pies, each	Mr Kipling	179	2.0	28.9	7.0	n/a
Raspberry & Cream Mivi, each	Lyons Maid	84.0	1.2	13.5	2.8	n/a
Raspberry & Redcurrant Creme Brulee	McVitie's	251	1.3	23.5	17.0	0.2

Product	*Brand*	*Calories kcal*	*Protein (g)*	*Carbo-hydrate (g)*	*Fat (g)*	*Dietary Fibre (g)*
Raspberry & Vanilla Swiss Roll	Lyons Bakeries	342	4.2	62.2	8.4	1.3
Raspberry Cheesecake	Young's	299	4.7	31.9	17.2	0.6
Raspberry Crisp	Mornflake	464	10.2	69.4	16.2	5.9
Raspberry Crusha	Burgess	112	Tr	27.8	nil	nil
Raspberry Flavour Jelly Crystals	Dietade	8.0	1.6	0.2	nil	nil
Raspberry Fromage Frais	St Ivel Shape	47.0	6.2	5.2	0.1	0.2
Raspberry Jam						
reduced sugar	Heinz Weight Watchers	125	0.6	30.3	0.3	1.3
sucrose free	Dietade	259	0.5	63.9	0.1	n/a
Raspberry Jelly, ready to eat	Rowntree	81.0	0.1	20.2	Tr	0.8
Raspberry Long Life Yogurt	St Ivel Prize	73.0	3.6	14.6	0.1	0.5
Raspberry Luxury Trifle	St Ivel	173	2.5	21.1	8.7	1.3

Raspberry Pavlova	McVitie's	297	2.5	45.0	11.9	Tr
Raspberry Preserve	Baxters	200	Tr	53.0	Tr	4.1
Raspberry Ready to Drink Carton	Robinsons	45.0	Tr	11.0	Tr	n/a
Raspberry Ripple Ice Cream	Fiesta	192	3.2	24.3	9.8	n/a
	Lyons Maid	114	1.6	19.0	3.5	n/a
Raspberry Ripple Mousse, each	Fiesta	90.0	2.0	11.4	4.0	n/a
Raspberry Swiss Roll	Lyons Bakeries	307	4.9	66.5	1.7	1.3
Raspberry Torte	Heinz Weight Watchers	132	3.1	19.3	4.7	0.5
	McVitie's	271	3.5	24.5	17.8	0.4
Raspberry Trifle per pack	St Ivel	153	1.5	24.9	5.4	0.5
	Boots Shapers	96.0	n/a	n/a	3.6	n/a
Raspberry Yogurt	St Ivel Shape	41.0	4.6	5.5	0.1	0.5
	Ski	94.0	5.1	17.0	1.1	nil
low fat	Holland & Barrett	83.0	5.4	13.5	0.8	0.5

All amounts given per 100g/100ml unless otherwise stated

Product	*Brand*	*Calories kcal*	*Protein (g)*	*Carbo-hydrate (g)*	*Fat (g)*	*Dietary Fibre (g)*
Ratatouille	Buitoni	45.0	1.3	5.3	1.9	0.9
Ravioli Bianche, as sold	Dolmio	200	9.6	29.7	4.7	n/a
Ravioli in Spicy Sauce	Heinz	69.0	3.0	12.3	0.9	0.6
Ravioli in Tomato Sauce	Heinz	74.0	2.8	13.1	1.1	0.8
Raw Cane Demerara Sugar	Tate & Lyle	400	0.1	99.2	nil	Tr
Ready Brek	Weetabix	359	12.0	59.9	8.4	8.4
Ready Cook Casserole	Itona	45.0	1.7	7.7	0.8	n/a
Ready Salted Crisps, per pack	Golden Wonder	155	1.9	12.0	11.0	1.3
Ready to Eat Prunes	Holland & Barrett	134	2.0	33.5	Tr	13.4
Real Cheese Nik Naks, per pack	Golden Wonder	188	2.2	17.7	12.1	0.3
Real Chocloate Chip Cookies	Heinz Weight Watchers	430	5.3	66.5	15.6	1.6

Real Chocolate Disney Mousse	Chambourcy	189	4.8	25.8	7.4	0.3
Real Fruit Pastilles, each	Trebor Bassett	17.4	0.1	4.1	nil	nil
Real Mayonnaise	Burgess	738	1.6	1.7	80.3	0.1
	Hellmanns	720	1.1	1.5	79.1	nil
Real Oyster Chinese Pouring Sauce	Sharwood	75.0	1.3	17.0	0.2	0.3
Red Butterfly Rice Pudding	Fussell's	91.0	3.2	16.0	1.6	0.2
Redcurrant Jelly	Burgess	129	0.6	30.9	nil	nil
	Colman's	368	0.7	90.0	Tr	n/a
Red Kidney Beans, boiled		103	8.4	17.4	0.5	9.0
canned		100	6.9	17.8	0.6	8.5
	Batchelors	103	8.4	21.1	0.5	5.0
	Holland & Barrett	100	6.9	17.8	0.6	6.2
Red Lentils: ***see Lentils***						
Red Pepper Chutney	Baxters	120	0.7	30.1	0.3	0.6

All amounts given per 100g/100ml unless otherwise stated

Product	*Brand*	*Calories kcal*	*Protein (g)*	*Carbo-hydrate (g)*	*Fat (g)*	*Dietary Fibre (g)*
Red Peppers: ***see Peppers***						
Red Salmon & Cucumber Sandwiches, per pack	Boots Shapers	235	n/a	n/a	n/a	n/a
Reduced Calorie Mayonnaise	Heinz Weight Watchers	275	1.5	7.6	26.5	nil
Reduced Fat Spreads: ***see individual brands/flavours***						
Reduced Salt Clover	Dairy Crest	388	7.1	n/a	39.9	n/a
Red Wine		68.0	0.2	0.3	nil	nil
Red Wine & Herb Sauce, as sold	Oxo	343	11.9	62.1	5.2	n/a
Red Wine & Herbs Ragu	Brooke Bond	84.0	1.9	12.1	2.8	n/a
Red Wine Casserole Sauce	Knorr	80.0	1.4	7.9	5.0	n/a
Red Wine Cook-In-Sauce	Homepride	47.0	0.5	8.5	1.2	n/a
Red Wine Ragu Sauce	Batchelors	84.0	1.9	12.1	2.8	n/a
Refreshers, each	Trebor Bassett	6.0	n/a	1.4	0.1	n/a

Revels	Mars	494	7.5	65.4	22.5	n/a
Rhubarb, stewed with sugar		48.0	0.9	11.5	0.1	1.2
stewed without sugar		7.0	0.9	0.7	0.1	1.3
canned in syrup		31.0	0.5	7.6	Tr	0.8
Rhubarb & Ginger Preserve	Baxters	210	Tr	53.0	Tr	1.7
Rhubarb Yogurt	St Ivel Shape	40.0	4.5	5.3	0.1	0.2
Ribena, undiluted		228	0.1	60.8	nil	nil
Rice, boiled						
brown		141	2.6	32.1	1.1	0.8
white		138	2.6	30.9	1.3	0.1
per packet, as served	Batchelors	842	20.9	165	10.6	12.0
Rice Krispies		369	6.1	89.7	0.9	0.7
	Kellogg's	370	6.0	85.0	0.9	0.7
Rice Pudding, canned		89.0	3.4	14.0	2.5	0.2
low fat, no added sugar	Heinz Weight Watchers	73.0	3.7	11.4	1.5	nil
Rich Beef Casserole Recipe Sauce	Knorr	38.0	1.2	8.2	0.3	n/a

All amounts given per 100g/100ml unless otherwise stated

Product	Brand	Calories kcal	Protein (g)	Carbo-hydrate (g)	Fat (g)	Dietary Fibre (g)
Rich Chocolate Slices, each	Mr Kipling	144	1.5	20.1	6.1	n/a
Rich Chocolate Tart	Mr Kipling	443	4.3	59.2	20.6	n/a
Rich Fruit Cake: ***see Fruit Cake***						
Rich Jamaican Spicy Barbecue Sauce	Lea & Perrins	159	1.2	35.4	1.4	n/a
Rich Redcurrant Drink, diluted	Robinsons	12.0	0.1	2.0	Tr	n/a
Rich Soy Chinese Pouring Sauce	Sharwood	48.0	4.6	7.5	Tr	0.3
Rich Tea Biscuits	McVitie's	470	6.7	74.2	15.7	2.3
	Peek Frean	440	7.2	7.2	13.7	0.2
Rich Tea Fingers	McVitie's	466	6.8	75.7	14.5	2.3
Rich Water Biscuits	Jacob's	436	9.8	69.2	13.3	2.8
Ricicles		381	4.3	95.7	0.5	0.4
	Kellogg's	380	4.0	89.0	0.6	0.5

Risotto, plain		224	3.0	34.4	9.3	0.4
Risotto Rice	Whitworths	324	7.0	77.8	0.6	0.2
Roast Beef & Gravy, per pack	Birds Eye Menu Master	95.0	16.0	3.0	2.0	Tr
Roast Beef in Gravy	Findus Dinner Supreme	84.0	14.0	2.4	2.1	nil
Roast Beef Platter, each	Birds Eye Menu Master	405	32.0	46.0	10.5	4.6
Roast Beef Salad Sandwiches, per pack	Boots Shapers	197	n/a	n/a	n/a	n/a
Roast Chicken & Back Bacon Sandwiches, per pack	Boots Shapers	222	n/a	n/a	n/a	n/a
Roast Chicken & Grape with Tarragon Mayonnaise Sandwiches, per pack	Boots Shapers	258	n/a	n/a	n/a	n/a
Roast Chicken Crisps, per pack	Golden Wonder	153	2.1	12.4	10.5	1.3

All amounts given per 100g/100ml unless otherwise stated

Product	*Brand*	*Calories kcal*	*Protein (g)*	*Carbo-hydrate (g)*	*Fat (g)*	*Dietary Fibre (g)*
Roast Chicken Platter, each	Birds Eye Menu Master	500	37.0	39.0	22.0	6.0
Roast Chicken Salad Roll, each	Boots Shapers	190	n/a	n/a	n/a	n/a
Roasted Cashew Nuts	Holland & Barrett	624	21.5	25.6	52.1	5.1
Roasted Salted Peanuts	Holland & Barrett	602	25.5	7.1	53.0	6.9
Roasted Sunflower Seeds in Shoyu Soy Sauce	Holland & Barrett	582	24.0	16.0	47.3	6.0
Roast Nut Tracker	Mars	516	10.0	52.8	29.4	n/a
Roast Turkey Platter, each	Birds Eye Menu Master	330	24.0	35.0	10.5	4.6
Roe						
cod, hard, fried		202	20.9	3.0	11.9	0.1
herring, soft, fried		244	21.1	4.7	15.8	N

Rogan Josh Classic Curry Sauce	Homepride	85.0	2.1	10.5	3.7	n/a
Rogan Josh Curry Cook-In-Sauce	Homepride	72.0	1.9	11.1	2.2	n/a
Rogan Josh Medium Curry Sauce	Colman's	45.0	1.5	n/a	0.6	n/a
	Sharwood	90.0	2.8	7.3	5.6	2.6
Rogan Josh Medium Curry Sauce mix, as sold	Sharwood	197	10.1	16.7	10.0	21.5
Rolls: ***see Bread Rolls***						
Rolo	Nestlé	482	62.7	5.2	23.4	n/a
Rolo Dessert	Chambourcy	245	3.2	30.9	12.1	0.2
Romano Pasta Choice Dry Mix, as sold	Crosse & Blackwell	385	12.3	65.7	7.1	3.5
Romany Biscuits	Jacob's	462	5.5	64.3	22.0	1.4
Rosehip Syrup, undiluted		232	Tr	61.9	nil	nil
Roses	Cadbury	480	4.7	62.6	23.6	n/a

All amounts given per 100g/100ml unless otherwise stated

Product	*Brand*	*Calories kcal*	*Protein (g)*	*Carbo-hydrate (g)*	*Fat (g)*	*Dietary Fibre (g)*
Rosé Wine		71.0	0.1	2.5	nil	nil
Rowntree Jelly Crystals, unsweetened, as sold, all flavours	Rowntree	225	56.4	nil	nil	nil
Royal Game Soup	Baxters	32.0	1.6	5.0	0.8	0.3
Royal Icing	Tate & Lyle	390	1.4	97.6	nil	nil
Royal Lemon Pie Filling Mix	Green's	147	4.7	27.6	4.7	n/a
Ruffle Bar	Cadbury	445	2.4	65.6	19.0	n/a
Rum: *see Spirits*						
Rum & Raisin Napoli	Lyons Maid	104	1.8	12.4	5.1	n/a
Rum Hot Chocolate, per pack	Boots Shapers	36.0	n/a	n/a	0.9	n/a
Rump Steak: *see Beef*						
Runner Beans, boiled		18.0	1.2	2.3	0.5	3.1
Rye Bread: *see Bread*						

Rye Crispbread		321	9.4	70.6	2.1	11.7
per slice	Boots Shapers	15.0	n/a	n/a	0.1	n/a
Rye Flour, whole		335	8.2	75.9	20.	11.7
Ryvita: ***see individual flavours***						

S

Product	Brand	Calories kcal	Protein (g)	Carbo-hydrate (g)	Fat (g)	Dietary Fibre (g)
Safflower Oil		899	Tr	nil	99.9	nil
Sage & Onion Stuffing		231	5.2	20.4	14.8	1.7
	Whitworths	398	5.7	73.6	9.0	1.9
Sage & Onion with Bacon Stuffing Mix	Knorr	420	10.5	64.7	13.2	n/a
Sago Pudding	Whitworths	355	0.2	94.0	0.2	nil
Saithe: ***see Coley***						
Salad Cream		348	1.5	16.7	31.0	N
reduced calorie		194	1.0	9.4	17.2	N
	Crosse &					

	Blackwell	370	1.6	15.5	33.0	0.5
light	Heinz	235	0.7	11.7	20.5	nil
Salad Mayonnaise	Burgess	579	2.4	8.1	59.2	nil
Salami		491	19.3	1.9	45.2	0.1
Salmon						
steamed, flesh only		197	20.1	nil	13.0	nil
canned		155	203.	nil	8.2	nil
smoked		142	25.4	nil	4.5	nil
Salmon & Asparagus with Tagliatelle	Findus Lean Cuisine	100	6.3	12.4	2.8	0.6
Salmon & Prawn Fricasee	Heinz Weight Watchers	74.0	6.0	6.5	2.4	0.5
Salmon & Shrimp Pâté	Shippams	182	15.3	2.4	12.4	n/a
Salmon Mornay	Heinz Weight Watchers	92.0	8.9	7.3	3.0	0.7
Salmon Pâté	Shippams	219	16.7	3.4	15.5	n/a
Salmon Rosti	Findus Lean Cuisine	80.0	4.6	9.9	2.3	0.9

Product	Brand	Calories kcal	Protein (g)	Carbo-hydrate (g)	Fat (g)	Dietary Fibre (g)
Salsa Lasagne	Napolina	83.0	3.1	8.6	4.0	n/a
Salsify, raw		27.0	1.3	10.2	0.3	3.2
boiled		23.0	1.1	8.6	0.4	3.5
Salt & Vinegar crisps, per pack	Golden Wonder	151	1.9	12.2	10.5	1.3
Salt & Vinegar Crunchy Fries, per pack	Golden Wonder	124	2.1	20.0	3.9	1.0
Salt & Vinegar Snakebites, per pack	Golden Wonder	106	1.2	12.4	5.7	0.2
Salt & Vinegar Supernaturals, per pack	Golden Wonder	89.0	1.1	10.8	4.6	0.2
Salted Cashew Nuts: *see Cashew Nuts*						
Salted Peanuts, per pack	Golden Wonder	232	9.9	11.6	16.6	2.7
Salted Rice Cakes	Holland & Barrett	376	8.5	77.2	3.1	7.5
Samosas, meat		593	5.1	17.9	56.1	1.2

vegetable		472	3.1	22.3	41.8	1.8
Sandwich Biscuits		513	5.0	69.2	25.9	N
Sandwich Cake Mixes: ***see individual flavours***						
Sandwich Cakes: ***see individual flavours***						
Sandwichmaker (Shippams): ***see individual flavours***						
Sandwich Spread	Heinz	221	1.3	25.3	12.7	0.8
Santa Bakewells, each	Mr Kipling	218	2.0	32.4	9.0	n/a
Sardine & Tomato Pâté	Shippams	156	18.0	3.0	8.0	n/a
Sardines						
canned in tomato sauce		177	17.8	0.5	11.6	Tr
canned in oil, drained		217	23.7	nil	13.6	nil
Satsumas, flesh only		36.0	0.9	8.5	0.1	1.3
Sauce à L'Orange Dry Mix, as sold	Crosse & Blackwell	367	4.5	71.7	6.9	0.5
Sauce Tartare: ***see Tartare Sauce***						
Saucy Beans	HP	73.0	5.4	12.2	0.6	7.3

Product	*Brand*	*Calories kcal*	*Protein (g)*	*Carbo-hydrate (g)*	*Fat (g)*	*Dietary Fibre (g)*
Sauerkraut		9.0	1.1	1.1	Tr	2.2
Sausage & Bean Casserole Simply Fix Dry Mix, as sold	Crosse & Blackwell	360	14.2	55.7	8.5	1.7
Sausage & Tomato Crisps, per pack	Golden Wonder	152	2.1	12.3	10.5	1.3
Sausage & Tomato Simply Fix Dry Mix, as sold	Crosse & Blackwell	355	11.9	56.7	8.3	2.5
Sausage Feast	Findus Dinner Supreme	166	6.2	15.0	9.0	2.1
Sausage Hotpot Toast Topper	Heinz	93.0	2.7	7.9	5.6	0.7
Sausage Hotpot with Pasta	Heinz	138	4.9	21.5	3.6	3.0
Sausage Pot Recipe Sauce Mix, as sold	Knorr	310	6.6	58.9	6.9	7.0
Sausage Rolls *flaky pastry*		477	7.1	32.3	36.4	1.2

short pastry		459	8.0	37.5	31.9	1.4
	Ross	289	11.1	19.4	19.3	0.8
Sausages, beef						
fried		269	12.9	14.9	18.0	0.7
grilled		265	13.0	15.2	17.3	0.7
Sausages, pork						
fried		317	13.8	11.0	24.5	0.7
grilled		318	13.3	11.5	24.6	0.7
low fat, fried		211	14.9	9.1	13.0	1.4
low fat, grilled		229	16.2	10.8	1.38	1.5
Sausages & Mash, per pack	Birds Eye Menu Master	505	16.0	50.0	27.0	2.8
Saveloy		262	9.9	10.1	20.5	N
Savoury Mince	Tyne Brand	86.0	9.8	13.4	7.3	0.6
Savoury Mince Recipe Sauce Mix, as sold	Knorr	286	8.4	52.2	6.2	4.0
Savoury Rice, cooked		142	2.9	26.3	3.5	1.4

Product	*Brand*	*Calories kcal*	*Protein (g)*	*Carbo-hydrate (g)*	*Fat (g)*	*Dietary Fibre (g)*
Savoury White Sauce Mix	Knorr	372	8.6	63.3	9.4	n/a
Scampi & Lemon Nik Naks, per pack	Golden Wonder	187	2.1	19.2	11.4	0.4
Scampi in Breadcrumbs, frozen, fried		316	12.2	28.9	17.6	N
Scoffins	Sunblest	292	7.1	49.8	7.1	1.8
Scones, fruit		316	7.3	52.9	9.8	N
plain		362	7.2	53.8	14.6	1.9
wholemeal		326	8.7	43.1	14.4	5.2
Scotch Broth	Baxters	39.0	1.2	6.4	1.1	0.8
	Campbell's	38.0	1.5	5.7	1.3	n/a
	Heinz	44.0	2.0	7.1	0.8	0.9
	Knorr	332	11.8	54.9	7.2	n/a
Scotch Eggs		251	12.0	13.1	17.1	N
Scotch Mince	Baxters	96.0	7.6	5.4	5.0	0.6
Scotch Orange Marmalade	Baxters	210	Tr	53.0	Tr	Tr

Scotch Pancakes		292	5.8	43.6	11.7	1.4
Scotch Shortbread Biscuit	Holland & Barrett	511	4.5	64.6	26.1	nil
Scotch Vegetable Soup	Baxters	26.0	0.6	5.2	0.5	0.8
Scotch Whisky: ***see Whisky***						
Scottish Haggis	Baxters	154	9.2	11.8	8.2	1.1
Scottish Lentil Soup	Crosse & Blackwell	44.0	2.6	6.2	1.0	1.0
Scottish Morning Rolls, each	Sunblest	122	4.5	22.6	1.5	0.8
Scottish Salmon Side	Young's	182	18.4	nil	12.0	nil
Scottish Salmon Slices	Young's	182	18.4	nil	12.0	nil
Scottish Square Bread	Mothers Pride	233	9.5	45.3	1.5	2.3
Scottish Vegetable Soup with Lentils	Heinz	47.0	2.9	7.1	0.8	1.0
Scotts Old Fashioned Porage Oats	Quaker	366	12.0	61.4	7.6	7.0

All amounts given per 100g/100ml unless otherwise stated

Product	Brand	Calories kcal	Protein (g)	Carbo-hydrate (g)	Fat (g)	Dietary Fibre (g)
Scotts Piper Oatmeal	Quaker	366	12.0	61.4	7.6	7.0
Scotts Porage Oats	Quaker	366	12.0	61.4	7.6	7.0
Scrambled Eggs: ***see Eggs***						
Seafood Bake with Broccoli	Heinz Weight Watchers	94.0	7.2	9.5	2.8	0.9
Seafood Cocktail	Lyons Seafoods	72.0	14.0	2.0	1.8	n/a
Seafood Crumble	Ross	197	8.7	11.3	13.2	0.5
Seafood Lasagne	Ross	117	7.2	10.7	5.3	1.0
Seafood Sauce	Colman's	395	0.9	13.0	37.0	n/a
Seafood Selection	Lyons Seafoods	81.0	14.9	1.3	2.3	n/a
	Young's	66.0	11.5	nil	2.2	nil
Seafood Sticks	Young's	97.0	10.7	14.1	0.1	nil
Secret	Nestlé	482	6.2	61.3	23.5	n/a
Seeded Burger Rolls, each	Sunblest	165	6.2	25.4	41.3	1.6

Seedless Raisins	Holland & Barrett	246	1.1	64.4	Tr	6.8
	Whitworths	307	2.6	73.3	0.4	2.0
Semi-skimmed Milk: *see Milk*						
Semolina Pudding	Whitworths	350	10.7	77.5	1.8	2.1
Semolina Whisk & Serve	Bird's	440	4.9	75.7	12.6	1.1
Sesame Oil		881	0.2	nil	99.7	nil
Sesame Ryvita, per slice	Ryvita	30.0	1.0	5.2	0.7	1.4
7 Up	Pepsi	44.0	nil	11.1	nil	n/a
Diet	Pepsi	1.7	nil	nil	nil	n/a
Seven Vegetable Premium Soup	Heinz	34.0	1.4	6.3	0.4	0.8
Shandy	Barr	30.0	n/a	7.4	Tr	Tr
Shandy Bass	Britvic	25.0	Tr	5.4	nil	n/a
Shape Milk Drink	St Ivel	44.0	3.2	5.2	101	Tr
Shapers (Boots): *see individual flavours*						

Product	Brand	Calories kcal	Protein (g)	Carbo-hydrate (g)	Fat (g)	Dietary Fibre (g)
Shepherd's Pie per pack	Ross	128	4.6	14.7	5.9	0.6
	Birds Eye Menu Master	220	11.0	25.0	8.5	1.9
Shepherd's Pie Filling	Tyne Brand	105	7.8	5.5	5.8	n/a
Shepherd's Pie Simply Fix Dry Mix, as sold	Crosse & Blackwell	295	13.4	45.9	6.4	1.8
Sherbert Lemons	Cravens	423	Tr	89.0	7.4	nil
Sherbet Dipper, each	Trebor Bassett	78.4	nil	18.9	nil	nil
Sherbet Fountain, each	Trebor Bassett	87.9	0.1	21.1	nil	nil
Sherbet Fruits	Cravens	423	Tr	89.0	7.4	nil
Sherbet Pips, each	Trebor Bassett	3.8	nil	0.9	nil	nil
Sherry						
dry		116	0.2	1.4	nil	nil
medium		118	0.1	3.6	nil	nil
sweet		136	0.3	6.9	nil	nil

Sherry Gateau	McVitie's	329	2.8	28.8	22.6	0.1
Shortbread		498	5.9	63.9	26.1	1.9
Shortcake Biscuits	Jacob's	464	5.4	67.0	21.2	1.8
Shortcake Snack	Cadbury	519	6.8	65.6	25.5	1.6
Shortcrust Pastry Mix	Whitworths	467	7.4	60.8	23.2	2.3
Shortcrust Pastry: *see Pastry*						
Short Grain Rice	Whitworths	361	6.5	86.8	1.0	2.4
Shorties	Cadbury	502	9.2	68.7	22.5	1.7
Shredded Cabbage	Ross	19.0	1.1	5.5	0.2	2.3
Shredded Wheat		325	10.6	68.3	3.0	9.8
Shreddies		331	10.0	74.1	1.5	9.5
Shrimps, frozen, without shells		73.0	16.5	nil	0.8	nil
canned, drained		94.0	20.8	nil	1.2	nil
Silverside, Sirloin: *see Beef*						
Silverskin Onions	Heinz	15.0	0.6	2.9	0.1	nil
Singles Cheese Slices	Kraft	295	19.0	2.7	23.0	nil

All amounts given per 100g/100ml unless otherwise stated

Product	*Brand*	*Calories kcal*	*Protein (g)*	*Carbo-hydrate (g)*	*Fat (g)*	*Dietary Fibre (g)*
Singles Light Cheese Slices	Kraft	200	21.0	5.0	11.0	nil
Skate, fried in batter		199	17.9	4.9	12.1	0.2
Skimmed Milk: *see Milk*						
Skittles	Mars	4.6	0.3	91.5	4.3	n/a
Slender Plan Drinks, etc.: *see Carnation Slender Plan…*						
Sliced Green Beans	Ross	31.0	1.8	7.6	0.2	2.2
Sliced Mushroom Ragu	Brooke Bond	77.0	1.9	11.8	2.7	n/a
Sliced Mushrooms, dried	Whitworths	223	16.5	40.0	1.0	22.9
Sliced Onions, dried	Whitworths	258	11.9	68.9	Tr	17.2
Slimline American Ginger Ale	Schweppes	0.7	n/a	Tr	n/a	n/a
Small Processed Peas	Batchelors	83.0	5.9	19.0	0.3	n/a
Smarties	Nestlé	459	5.4	71.1	17.0	n/a
Smatana	Raines	130	4.7	5.6	10.0	n/a

Smoked Fish with Pasta Bows	Heinz Weight Watchers	85.0	6.6	10.1	2.0	0.7
Smoked Haddock Cutlets	Ross	77.0	17.8	nil	0.6	nil
Smoked Haddock Fillets with Butter	Birds Eye Captain's Table	93.0	19.0	nil	1.9	nil
Smoked Ham & Egg Sandwiches, per pack	Boots Shapers	278	n/a	n/a	n/a	n/a
Smoked Ham & Lettuce Four Pack Selection Sandwiches, per pack	Boots Shapers	290	n/a	n/a	n/a	n/a
Smoked Ham & Mushroom Pizza, deep pan	McCain	183	10.7	27.0	4.3	n/a
Smoked Ham, Cheese & Tomato with Pickle Sandwiches, per pack	Boots Shapers	191	n/a	n/a	n/a	n/a
Smoked Ham Salad Sandwiches, per pack	Boots Shapers	186	n/a	n/a	n/a	n/a

Product	*Brand*	*Calories kcal*	*Protein (g)*	*Carbo-hydrate (g)*	*Fat (g)*	*Dietary Fibre (g)*
Smoked Ham, Soft Cheese & Pineapple Sandwiches, per pack	Boots Shapers	188	n/a	n/a	n/a	n/a
Smoked Turkey & Bacon with Guacamole & Fresh Coriander Sandwiches, per pack	Boots Shapers	196	n/a	n/a	n/a	n/a
Smokey Barbecue Sauce	Heinz	89.0	1.2	20.5	0.2	0.7
Smoky Bacon & Tomato Snack-A-Soup Special, per sachet	Batchelors	165	4.8	29.3	3.1	3.2
Smoky Bacon Crisps, per pack	Golden Wonder	152	2.0	12.4	10.5	1.3
Smooth & Creamy Mayonnaise Style Dressing	Kraft	122	0.6	7.8	9.7	0.4
Smooth Hot Chocolate	Boots Shapers	37.0	n/a	n/a	0.9	n/a

Smooth Peanut Butter	Holland & Barrett	585	24.0	29.0	41.0	nil
	Sunpat	620	25.8	14.5	50.9	6.5
Snickers	Mars	510	10.2	54.1	26.4	n/a
Snowballs	Tunnock's	388	3.9	47.0	21.8	n/a
Snow Chocs Cakes	Mr Kipling	120	1.7	15.0	5.6	n/a
Soft Brown Rolls	Heinz Weight Watchers	193	8.9	36.1	1.5	4.7
Soft Cheese Spread						
with Garlic & Herbs	St Ivel Shape	106	10.8	9.8	2.6	nil
with Smoked Ham	St Ivel Shape	107	11.0	9.4	2.8	nil
Soft Cheese						
with Garlic & Herbs, 28g/1oz	Primula	83.0	n/a	n/a	n/a	n/a
with Red Pepper, 28g/1oz	Primula	80.0	n/a	n/a	n/a	n/a
Soft Fruit Centres	Cravens	386	Tr	96.4	nil	nil
Softmints, each	Trebor Bassett	16.0	n/a	3.5	0.2	n/a

Product	*Brand*	*Calories kcal*	*Protein (g)*	*Carbo-hydrate (g)*	*Fat (g)*	*Dietary Fibre (g)*
Soft White Rolls	Heinz Weight Watchers	202	8.7	39.2	1.2	2.7
Soft Wholemeal Bread	Hovis	215	10.5	37.9	2.4	7.2
Sole: ***see Lemon Sole***						
Soup: ***see individual flavours***						
Soup & Broth Mix	Whitworths	332	14.1	70.2	1.4	8.6
Soupe au Pistou	Baxters	30.0	1.0	6.5	0.3	1.2
Sour Cream & Chive Crinkle Crisps, per pack	Boots Shapers	93.0	n/a	n/a	4.4	n/a
Sour Cream & Chives Wheat Crunchies, per pack	Golden Wonder	180	3.6	20.3	9.3	1.0
Southern Fried Chicken, per piece	Birds Eye Steakhouse	265	15.0	13.0	17.0	1.4
Southern Fries Savoury Spirals	McCain	231	2.7	27.3	12.3	2.3

Southern Fries Savoury Straight Cut	McCain	179	2.7	26.4	6.8	n/a
Southern Fries Savoury Wedges	McCain	151	7.2	24.8	5.2	n/a
Southern Fries Spicy Lattice	McCain	206	2.8	25.8	10.2	n/a
Soya Bean Curd: *see Tofu*						
Soya Beans, boiled		141	14.0	5.1	7.3	6.1
Soya Chunks Flavoured	Holland & Barrett	250	50.5	11.0	0.8	5.1
Unflavoured	Holland & Barrett	250	50.5	11.0	0.8	5.1
Soya Curd: *see Tofu*						
Soya Flour						
full fat		447	36.8	23.5	23.5	11.2
low fat		352	45.3	28.2	7.2	13.5
Soya Milk, plain		32.0	2.9	0.8	1.9	nil
flavoured		40.0	2.8	3.6	1.7	nil

All amounts given per 100g/100ml unless otherwise stated

Product	*Brand*	*Calories kcal*	*Protein (g)*	*Carbo-hydrate (g)*	*Fat (g)*	*Dietary Fibre (g)*
Soya Mince Flavoured	Holland & Barrett	250	50.5	11.0	0.8	5.0
Unflavoured	Holland & Barrett	250	51.5	11.0	0.8	5.1
Soy & Five Spice Sauce	Lea & Perrins	98.0	1.4	21.7	0.5	n/a
Soy & Garlic Sauce	Lea & Perrins	88.0	0.9	19.8	0.6	n/a
Soya Oil		899	Tr	nil	99.9	nil
Soya Yogurt: *see Yogurt*						
Soy Sauce, dark, thick		64.0	8.7	8.3	nil	nil
Spaghetti, cooked						
white		104	3.6	22.2	0.7	1.2
wholemeal		113	4.7	23.2	0.9	3.5
Spaghetti Bolognese	Heinz	97.0	3.7	14.7	2.6	1.1
	Heinz Weight Watchers Heinz Lunch	80.0	5.3	10.8	1.8	0.9

	Bowl	110	4.7	12.8	4.5	0.8
per pack	Birds Eye Menu Master	450	21.0	58.0	15.0	3.8
low calorie	Findus Lean Cuisine	84.0	5.5	11.0	1.9	1.1
Spaghetti Bolognese Microchef Snack	Batchelors	63.0	4.5	8.5	1.1	n/a
Spaghetti Bolognese Sauce	Campbell's	62.0	2.7	9.4	1.5	n/a
Spaghetti Bolognese Sauce Mix, as sold	Colman's	313	9.5	64.0	1.1	n/a
Spaghetti Bolognese Sauce with Mushrooms	Campbell's	66.0	2.6	10.4	1.6	n/a
Spaghetti Bolognese Sauce with Onions & Garlic	Campbell's	66.0	2.6	10.3	106	n/a
Spaghetti Bolognese Simply Fix Dry Mix, as sold	Crosse & Blackwell	320	11.6	51.8	5.5	3.2
Spaghetti Hoops	Heinz	61.0	1.9	12.6	0.4	0.8

All amounts given per 100g/100ml unless otherwise stated

Product	*Brand*	*Calories kcal*	*Protein (g)*	*Carbo-hydrate (g)*	*Fat (g)*	*Dietary Fibre (g)*
Spaghetti Hoops with Hotdogs	Heinz	90.0	2.9	11.1	3.7	0.5
Spaghetti in Tomato Sauce no added sugar	Heinz	64.0	1.7	13.5	0.4	0.7
	Heinz Weight Watchers	51.0	1.7	10.1	0.4	0.7
Spaghetti Sauce Mix	Knorr	355	7.9	65.5	6.8	n/a
Spaghetti Shapes	Heinz Noodle Doodles	69.0	2.1	13.8	0.6	0.9
	Heinz Super Mario	67.0	2.3	13.5	0.4	0.8
Spaghetti with Sausages in Tomato Sauce	Heinz	108	3.8	12.5	4.7	0.7
Spaghetti with Vitamins (straight/hoops)	Crosse & Blackwell	63.0	1.8	13.0	0.4	0.4
Spanish Chicken Tonight Sauce	Batchelors	60.0	1.0	16.0	5.7	n/a

Spare Rib Nik Naks, per pack	Golden Wonder	195	2.1	18.4	12.6	0.4
Spearmint Chewing Gum	Wrigley	288	nil	71.0	nil	nil
Special K		377	15.3	81.7	1.0	2.0
	Kellogg's	370	15.0	75.0	1.0	2.5
Special Recipe Muesli	Jordans	360	10.4	57.2	10.0	9.0
Special Rice Mix	Ross	59.0	2.6	13.5	0.4	2.0
Special Soft Spread	Kraft	635	0.3	1.0	70.0	nil
Special Vegetable Mix	Ross	46.0	3.0	11.2	0.3	3.5
Spiced Basmati Rice	Sharwood	365	9.3	73.2	1.7	nil
Spiced Fruit Chutney	Baxters	131	0.6	34.1	Tr	1.1
Spiced Poppadums	Sharwood	281	20.4	45.6	1.9	10.3
Spicy Bean & Vegetable Wholesome Soup	Heinz Weight Watchers	30.0	1.3	5.8	0.2	1.1
Spicy Bean Salad	Batchelors	115	7.5	22.5	1.4	4.5
Spicy Beef Pasta Twists	Heinz	85.0	3.8	12.3	2.3	0.8

All amounts given per 100g/100ml unless otherwise stated

Product	*Brand*	*Calories kcal*	*Protein (g)*	*Carbo-hydrate (g)*	*Fat (g)*	*Dietary Fibre (g)*
Spicy Beef Stew	Tyne Brand	106	7.5	8.1	5.1	n/a
Spicy Chicken Creole with Rice	Findus Lean Cuisine	100	7.0	14.9	1.4	1.3
Spicy Chicken Deep South Recipe Sauce	Homepride	80.0	1.0	17.0	0.7	n/a
Spicy Chicken Pot Light	Golden Wonder	322	15.3	59.5	2.5	n/a
Spicy Crunchy Fries, per pack	Golden Wonder	134	2.0	18.2	5.7	0.9
Spicy Curry Pot Noodle	Golden Wonder	405	11.1	64.2	11.5	n/a
Spicy Parsnip Soup	Baxters	49.0	2.3	5.4	2.2	1.4
Spicy Pepper Sauce	Heinz	81.0	1.9	17.2	0.6	0.5
Spicy Sandwich Spread	Heinz	214	1.3	24.0	12.6	0.8
Spicy Szechuan Chicken Pots of the World	Golden Wonder	398	11.1	57.7	13.6	n/a
Spicy Tomato Pizza Topping	Napolina	78.0	1.4	7.2	5.0	n/a

Spicy Tomato Ragu	Brooke Bond	84.0	2.0	13.0	3.0	n/a
Spicy Tomato Sauce	HP	121	1.6	26.5	1.0	n/a
Spicy Tomato Wheat Crunchies, per pack	Golden Wonder	180	3.6	20.3	9.3	1.0
Spicy Tomato with Beef Pasta Parcels Soup	Heinz	67.0	2.4	10.0	1.9	1.2
Spicy Vegetable Snack-A-Soup Special, per sachet	Batchelors	190	4.2	30.4	5.7	2.1
Spinach, raw		25.0	2.8	1.6	0.8	2.1
boiled		19.0	2.2	0.8	0.8	2.1
frozen, boiled		21.0	3.1	0.5	0.8	2.1
Spinach & Lentil Spread, per pack	Boots Shapers	87.0	n/a	n/a	3.2	n/a
Spira	Cadbury	525	7.8	56.8	29.4	n/a
Spiral Oven Fries	McCain	196	2.0	31.4	9.2	n/a
Spirits, 40% volume (mean of brandy, gin, rum, vodka, whisky)		222	Tr	Tr	nil	nil

All amounts given per 100g/100ml unless otherwise stated

Product	Brand	Calories kcal	Protein (g)	Carbo-hydrate (g)	Fat (g)	Dietary Fibre (g)
Split Peas, dried, boiled		126	8.3	22.7	0.9	2.7
Sponge Cake		459	6.4	52.4	26.3	0.9
fatless		294	10.1	53.0	6.1	0.9
jam filled		302	4.2	64.2	4.9	1.8
with butter icing		490	4.5	52.4	30.6	0.6
Sponge Cake Mixes: *see individual flavours*						
Sponge Finger Biscuits	Huntley & Palmer	400	7.4	90.6	4.0	1.3
Sponge Pudding		340	5.8	45.3	16.3	1.1
Sport Biscuits	McVitie's	516	6.4	62.9	26.5	1.7
Spotted Dick	McVitie's	357	5.7	51.2	15.0	2.3
Spotted Dick Microbake Mix	Homepride	308	4.0	55.5	8.0	n/a
Spreads, Dairy, Low Fat, etc.: *see individual brands/flavours*						
Spring Garden Vegetable Reduced Calorie Soup	Batchelors	24.0	0.9	3.0	1.0	n/a

Spring Garden Vegetable Soup	Batchelors	40.0	1.0	4.5	2.0	n/a
Spring Greens, raw		33.0	3.0	3.1	1.0	3.4
boiled		20.0	1.9	1.6	0.7	0.7
Spring Onion & Garlic Stir & Serve Sauce	Knorr	504	10.0	46.3	31.0	n/a
Spring Onion Crisps, per pack	Golden Wonder	153	2.0	12.6	10.5	1.3
Spring Onions, bulbs & tops, raw		23.0	2.0	3.0	0.5	1.5
Spring Vegetable Low Calorie Soup	Knorr	309	11.0	65.3	0.4	n/a
Spring Vegetable Soup	Heinz	31.0	0.8	6.6	0.2	0.8
Sprouts: ***see Brussels Sprouts***						
Spry Crisp 'n' Dry, solid/oil	Van Den Berghs	900	nil	nil	100	n/a
Squash: ***see Courgettes***						
Starbar	Cadbury	490	10.7	49.0	27.9	n/a

Product	*Brand*	*Calories kcal*	*Protein (g)*	*Carbo-hydrate (g)*	*Fat (g)*	*Dietary Fibre (g)*
Steak: ***see Beef***						
Steak & Kidney Pie, individual		323	9.1	25.6	21.2	0.9
	Ross	232	8.5	22.4	12.4	0.9
pastry top only		286	15.2	15.9	18.4	0.6
Steak & Onion Crisps, per pack	Golden Wonder	152	2.0	12.2	10.6	1.2
Steak in Red Wine Platter, per meal	Birds Eye Healthy Options	330	27.0	37.0	8.00	3.3
Stem Ginger Cookies	Heinz Weight Watchers	399	5.0	64.5	13.4	1.4
Stew: ***see individual flavours***						
Stewed Steak with Gravy, canned		176	14.8	1.0	1.25	Tr
Still Lemonade Fruit Burst	Del Monte	42.0	0.2	10.6	Tr	n/a
Stilton & Celery Soup	Baxters	83.0	3.5	4.3	5.4	0.2
Stilton, blue		411	22.7	0.1	35.5	nil

Stir Fry Chinese Style Rice	Uncle Ben's	143	2.7	26.3	3.0	n/a
Stir Fry Noodles	Sharwood	358	7.3	79.6	1.2	3.7
Stock Cubes: ***see individual flavours***						
Stollen Slices, each	Mr Kipling	210	2.4	30.3	8.5	n/a
Stoneground Bread	Hovis	220	11.2	38.9	2.3	6.8
Stoneground Wholemeal Baps, each	Allinson	139	5.9	22.4	2.9	3.6
Stoneground Wholemeal Bread, 100%	Allinson	220	9.7	38.5	3.0	6.5
Stork Light Blend Spread	Van Den Berghs	542	0.1	0.4	60.0	nil
Stork Margarine	Van Den Berghs	731	0.1	0.4	81.0	nil
Stork Special Blend Margarine	Van Den Berghs	731	0.1	0.4	81.0	nil
Stout, bottled		37.0	0.3	4.2	Tr	nil
extra		39.0	0.3	2.1	Tr	nil
Straight Cut Chips	McCain	132	2.4	21.9	3.9	n/a
Straight Microchips	McCain	200	3.5	24.7	10.5	n/a

All amounts given per 100g/100ml unless otherwise stated

Product	*Brand*	*Calories kcal*	*Protein (g)*	*Carbo-hydrate (g)*	*Fat (g)*	*Dietary Fibre (g)*
Straight Oven Chips	McCain	154	1.9	26.9	4.3	n/a
Strawberries, raw		27.0	0.8	6.0	0.1	1.1
canned in syrup		65.0	0.5	16.9	Tr	0.7
Strawberries & Cream Premium Ice Cream	Heinz Weight Watchers	117	2.9	15.7	4.3	0.2
Strawberry & Apple Pies	Lyons Bakeries	381	3.2	56.7	15.6	1.2
Strawberry & Coconut Yogurt	St Ivel Shape	41.0	4.5	5.6	0.1	0.2
Strawberry & Cream Cheesecake	Young's	296	4.6	31.9	16.9	0.2
Strawberry & Cream Mivi, each	Lyons Maid	83.0	1.0	13.4	2.7	n/a
Strawberry & Cream Torte	Heinz Weight Watchers	14.0	3.1	21.9	4.4	0.4
Strawberry & Vanilla Fromage Frais	St Ivel Shape	50.0	6.2	6.0	0.1	0.2

Strawberry & Vanilla Sundae, per pack	Boots Shapers	121	n/a	n/a	4.2	n/a
Strawberry & Vanilla Yogurt	St Ivel Shape	41.0	4.5	5.6	0.1	0.2
Strawberry Bio Splitpot, per pack	Boots Shapers	79.0	n/a	n/a	0.2	n/a
Strawberry Blancmange Powder, as sold	Brown & Polson	342	0.6	83.0	0.7	n/a
Strawberry Bonbons, each	Trebor Bassett	28.0	nil	5.8	nil	nil
Strawberry Cheesecake	Green's/ Homepride	258	3.0	31.5	12.0	n/a
	Heinz Weight Watchers	160	4.3	26.1	4.0	0.4
	McVitie's	390	4.9	31.9	22.7	0.4
Strawberry Country Crisp	Jordans	435	7.4	64.5	16.4	8.0
Strawberry Cream Cake	McVitie's	271	3.2	37.4	12.8	1.6
Strawberry Creme de Creme, each	Lyons Maid	174	2.3	26.0	7.2	n/a

Product	*Brand*	*Calories kcal*	*Protein (g)*	*Carbo-hydrate (g)*	*Fat (g)*	*Dietary Fibre (g)*
Strawberry Creme Yogurt	St Ivel Shape	41.0	4.5	5.6	0.1	0.2
Strawberry Crisp	Mornflake	464	10.2	69.4	16.2	5.9
Strawberry Crusha	Burgess	111	Tr	27.8	nil	nil
Strawberry Dairy Ice Cream	Heinz Weight Watchers	132	3.0	16.8	5.5	nil
		101	2.8	15.9	3.0	n/a
Strawberry Dessert Pot	Ambrosia					
Strawberry Devonshire Cheesecake	St Ivel	262	4.9	28.9	14.3	1.3
Strawberry Drinking Yoghurt, low fat, per pack	Boots Shapers	80.0	n/a	n/a	Tr	n/a
Strawberry Flavour Jelly Crystals	Dietade	7.0	1.5	0.1	nil	nil
Strawberry Fromage Frais	St Ivel Shape	50.0	6.2	5.6	0.1	0.2
	Ski	123	6.1	14.0	4.8	n/a
Strawberry Fruit Sundae, per pack	Boots Shapers	80.0	n/a	n/a	4.0	n/a

Strawberry Gateau	McVitie's	274	2.3	30.4	16.4	1.0
	St Ivel	269	2.3	27.9	16.6	0.6
Strawberry Ice Cream	Fiesta	176	3.8	18.5	10.2	n/a
	Lyons Maid	84.0	1.7	10.5	3.8	n/a
per pack	Boots Shapers	102	n/a	n/a	3.9	n/a
Strawberry Jam reduced sugar	Heinz Weight Watchers	126	0.4	31.0	0.1	0.6
	Holland & Barrett	140	0.5	36.0	nil	nil
sucrose free	Dietade	257	0.3	63.8	Tr	n/a
Strawberry Jam Mini Rolls, each	Cadbury	117	1.4	17.7	4.5	n/a
Strawberry Jam Sponge Pudding	Heinz	285	2.8	46.3	9.8	0.7
Strawberry Jelly, ready to eat	Rowntree	67.0	0.1	16.7	Tr	0.5
Strawberry King Cone, each	Lyons Maid	186	2.0	28.9	6.8	n/a

All amounts given per 100g/100ml unless otherwise stated

Product	*Brand*	*Calories kcal*	*Protein (g)*	*Carbo-hydrate (g)*	*Fat (g)*	*Dietary Fibre (g)*
Strawberry Lightly Whipped Yogurt	St Ivel Prize	135	4.3	15.2	6.4	nil
Strawberry Long Life Yogurt	St Ivel Prize	71.0	3.4	14.3	0.1	0.4
Strawberry Luxury Trifle	St Ivel	167	2.5	21.0	8.1	0.6
Strawberry Mousse, each	Fiesta	75.0	1.7	9.0	3.6	n/a
Strawberry Mr Men, each	Lyons Maid	28.0	nil	7.0	nil	n/a
Strawberry Napoli	Lyons Maid	102	1.8	12.2	5.1	n/a
Strawberry Nesquik	Nestlé	391	nil	96.7	0.5	nil
made up with whole milk	Nestlé	168	6.8	18.8	3.7	n/a
with semi-skimmed milk	Nestlé	131	6.8	18.8	3.7	n/a
ready to drink	Nestlé	68.0	3.2	10.0	1.7	nil
Strawberry Pavlova	McVitie's	330	2.3	32.7	21.1	nil
Strawberry Preserve	Baxters	210	Tr	53.0	Tr	1.4
Strawberry Summer Rolls	Lyons Bakeries	348	4.2	65.2	7.4	1.0
Strawberry Sundaes, each	Mr Kipling	194	1.4	29.4	7.9	n/a

Strawberry Surprise Hot Chocolate, per pack	Boots Shapers	40.0	n/a	n/a	0.9	n/a
Strawberry Toppit, each	Nestlé	92.0	1.2	18.9	1.3	n/a
Strawberry Trifle	St Ivel	149	1.5	24.0	5.4	0.3
	Young's	142	1.4	26.6	3.7	0.2
Strawberry Twinpot Yogurt	St Ivel Shape	59.0	4.4	8.3	1.0	0.4
Strawberry Yogurt per pack	St Ivel Shape	41.0	4.5	5.6	0.1	0.2
	Boots Shapers	53.0	n/a	n/a	0.1	n/a
Strawberry Yogurt Mousse, per pack	Boots Shapers	55.0	n/a	n/a	1.5	n/a
Straw Mushroom: *see Mushrooms*						
Strike Cola	Barr	38.0	n/a	9.4	Tr	Tr
Stringfellows Oven Fries	McCain	180	2.7	26.0	7.2	n/a
Stroganoff Pour Over Sauce	Baxters	107	3.0	8.3	6.7	0.1
Strollers	Cadbury	448	6.6	65.8	21.5	n/a

All amounts given per 100g/100ml unless otherwise stated

Product	Brand	Calories kcal	Protein (g)	Carbo-hydrate (g)	Fat (g)	Dietary Fibre (g)
Strong Ale		72.0	0.7	6.1	Tr	nil
Strongbow White Cider	H P Bulmer	52.4	n/a	n/a	n/a	n/a
Stuffed Pork Roll	Tyne Brand	147	4.5	9.6	7.0	n/a
Stuffed Turkey Roll	Tyne Brand	150	13.0	7.8	7.4	n/a
Stuffing Mixes: *see individual flavours*						
Suet, shredded		826	Tr	12.1	86.7	0.5
Sugar: *see Caster, Granulated, etc.*						
Sugar Frosted Cornflakes	Sunblest	385	6.3	88.0	0.9	1.1
Sugar Puffs		324	5.9	84.5	0.8	3.2
	Quaker	387	6.5	86.5	1.0	3.0
Sugared Almonds	Cravens	430	4.4	78.1	11.1	2.3
Sultana & Apple Crunch	Mornflake	404	11.0	63.0	12.0	7.5
Sultana & Cinnamon Cookies	Heinz Weight Watchers	401	5.0	67.7	12.2	1.8

Sultana & Syrup Pancakes	Sunblest	275	5.8	48.9	6.2	2.2
Sultana Bran		303	8.5	67.8	1.6	10.0
	Kellogg's	310	9.0	64.0	2.0	11.0
Sultanas		275	2.7	69.4	0.4	2.0
	Holland & Barrett	250	1.8	64.7	Tr	7.0
Summer County Reduced Fat Spread	Van Den Berghs	542	0.1	0.4	60.0	nil
Summer Fruit Drink	Rowntree	48.0	Tr	11.7	Tr	nil
Summer Fruit Layered Desert, per pack	Boots Shapers	90.0	n/a	n/a	2.4	n/a
Summer Fruits Crumble	Jacob's	483	6.0	63.4	22.7	3.0
Summer Fruits Special R, diluted	Robinsons	8.0	0.1	0.9	Tr	n/a
Summer Gateau	Mr Kipling	413	4.8	57.4	17.2	n/a
Sunblest Bread, etc.: *see individual flavours*						
Sunflower Seed Oil		899	Tr	nil	99.9	nil

Product	*Brand*	*Calories kcal*	*Protein (g)*	*Carbo-hydrate (g)*	*Fat (g)*	*Dietary Fibre (g)*
Sunflower Seeds	Holland & Barrett	582	24.0	16.0	47.3	6.0
Sunflower Spread	Vitalite	685	0.2	1.3	75.0	nil
reduced fat	Vitalite	510	0.2	1.3	56.0	nil
Sunfruit Juice, per pack	Boots Shapers	41.0	n/a	n/a	Tr	n/a
Sunmalt Malt Loaf	Sunblest	265	9.7	51.7	2.2	5.3
Super Chicken Low Calorie Soup	Knorr	308	13.1	55.8	3.6	n/a
Super Chicken Noodle Quick Soup	Knorr	343	8.2	65.9	5.2	n/a
Super Chicken Noodle Soup	Knorr	350	14.2	57.3	7.1	n/a
Super Deluxe Deep Pan Pizza	McCain	195	9.9	28.0	5.5	n/a
Supernoodles (Batchelors): ***see individual flavours***						
Super Value Vanilla Ice Cream	Fiesta	154	3.4	20.4	7.1	n/a
Supreme Chicken Noodle Packet Soup, as served	Batchelors	204	11.5	38.5	2.1	4.1

Swede, boiled		11.0	0.3	2.3	0.1	0.7
Swedish Cauliflower & Broccoli Soup of the World	Knorr	458	6.5	43.9	28.5	n/a
Sweet & Sour Bistro Break	HP	119	5.2	18.6	2.0	0.4
Sweet & Sour Casserole Recipe Sauce	Knorr	58.0	0.9	14.5	Tr	n/a
Sweet & Sour Chicken	Vesta	108	2.8	22.8	1.2	n/a
per single serving	Vesta	525	14.2	104.3	5.7	n/a
Sweet & Sour Chicken Potato Topper	Heinz Weight Watchers	64.0	3.7	9.3	1.3	0.9
Sweet & Sour Chicken Pot Noodle	Golden Wonder	420	11.2	61.2	14.4	n/a
Sweet & Sour Chicken Simply Fix Dry Mix, as sold	Crosse & Blackwell	330	5.2	56.2	7.6	0.7
Sweet & Sour Chicken with Rice	Heinz Weight Watchers	94.0	5.7	14.2	1.6	0.2
per pack	Birds Eye Menu Master	400	20.4	72.0	3.5	1.5

All amounts given per 100g/100ml unless otherwise stated

Product	*Brand*	*Calories kcal*	*Protein (g)*	*Carbo-hydrate (g)*	*Fat (g)*	*Dietary Fibre (g)*
Sweet & Sour Cook-In-Sauce	Homepride	82.0	0.4	7.8	0.2	n/a
Sweet & Sour King Prawns	Ross	195	6.6	15.1	12.2	0.4
Sweet & Sour Pork Stir Fry Dry Mix, as sold	Crosse & Blackwell	370	2.7	81.5	3.1	0.4
Sweet & Sour Pork with Rice	Heinz	104	4.3	16.1	2.5	0.7
Sweet & Sour Sauce	Burgess	150	0.6	35.2	Tr	0.2
	HP	146	0.9	33.5	0.8	n/a
Sweet & Sour Sauce & Vegetable Stir Fry	Uncle Ben's	94.0	0.4	23.2	Tr	n/a
Sweet 'n' Sour Sauce Mix, dry, as sold	Colman's	334	3.3	78.0	0.1	n/a
Sweet & Sour Stir Fry Sauce	Homepride	100	0.5	24.9	0.1	n/a
	Sharwood	84.0	0.6	19.9	2.2	1.1
	Uncle Ben's	104	0.3	25.7	Tr	n/a
Sweet & Sour Vegetables	Heinz Weight Watchers	70.0	2.4	14.0	0.4	1.1

Sweetbread, lamb, fried		230	19.4	5.6	14.6	0.1
Sweet Chilli Chinese Pouring Sauce	Sharwood	187	0.6	44.4	0.8	1.5
Sweetcorn						
baby, fresh/frozen, boiled		24.0	2.5	2.7	0.4	2.0
baby, canned		23.0	2.9	2.0	0.4	1.5
kernels, boiled		111	4.2	19.6	2.3	2.2
kernels, canned		122	2.9	26.6	1.2	1.4
on-the-cob, boiled		66.0	2.5	11.6	1.4	1.3
Sweetcorn & Red Pepper Sandwich Spread	Heinz	203	2.1	22.4	11.7	1.0
Sweet Corn, Peas & Carrots, 1oz/28g	Birds Eye	18.0	1.0	3.0	0.2	0.8
Sweet Peanuts, each	Trebor Bassett	27.2	0.1	5.1	0.6	nil
Sweet Pepper Pasta Choice Dry Mix, as sold	Crosse & Blackwell	355	13.4	66.3	4.0	4.3
Sweet Peppers with Chilli Sauce	Lea & Perrins	73.0	1.3	15.8	0.7	n/a

All amounts given per 100g/100ml unless otherwise stated

Product	Brand	Calories kcal	Protein (g)	Carbo-hydrate (g)	Fat (g)	Dietary Fibre (g)
Sweet Pickle	Burgess	167	0.9	39.3	Tr	1.9
	Heinz Ploughman's	114	0.8	27.3	0.2	1.0
Sweet Potato, boiled		84.0	1.1	20.5	0.3	2.3
Swiss Gateau	Cadbury	417	5.4	56.5	18.8	n/a
Swiss Rolls, Chocolate, individual		337	4.3	58.1	11.3	N
Swiss Style Chocolate Dessert	Chambourcy	256	4.1	29.4	13.6	0.1
Syrup, Golden		298	0.3	79.0	nil	nil
Szechuan Chilli Sauce & Vegetable Stir Fry	Uncle Ben's	88.0	1.2	11.1	4.4	n/a

T

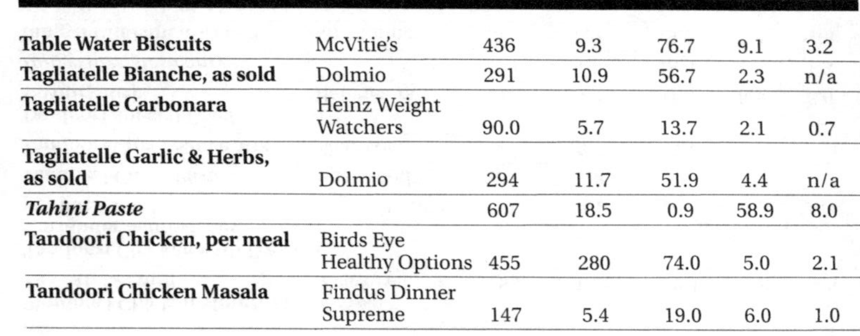

Table Water Biscuits	McVitie's	436	9.3	76.7	9.1	3.2
Tagliatelle Bianche, as sold	Dolmio	291	10.9	56.7	2.3	n/a
Tagliatelle Carbonara	Heinz Weight Watchers	90.0	5.7	13.7	2.1	0.7
Tagliatelle Garlic & Herbs, as sold	Dolmio	294	11.7	51.9	4.4	n/a
Tahini Paste		607	18.5	0.9	58.9	8.0
Tandoori Chicken, per meal	Birds Eye Healthy Options	455	280	74.0	5.0	2.1
Tandoori Chicken Masala	Findus Dinner Supreme	147	5.4	19.0	6.0	1.0

All amounts given per 100g/100ml unless otherwise stated

Product	*Brand*	*Calories kcal*	*Protein (g)*	*Carbo-hydrate (g)*	*Fat (g)*	*Dietary Fibre (g)*
Tandoori Chicken Simply Fix Dry Mix, as sold	Crosse & Blackwell	265	13.1	32.1	7.8	9.5
Tandoori Chicken with Fresh Coriander Sandwiches, per pack	Boots Shapers	193	n/a	n/a	n/a	n/a
Tandoori Curry Paste	Sharwood	237	5.0	9.1	20.1	4.7
Tandoori Curry Sauce Mix	Sharwood	221	9.5	30.1	7.0	11.1
Tandoori Special Fried Savoury Rice	Batchelors	482	10.9	91.5	8.1	6.0
Tangerines, flesh only		35.0	1.0	18.0	1.5	1.3
Tangy Fruit Fancies, each	Mr Kipling	107	0.6	19.6	2.8	n/a
Tangy Sandwich Pickle	Heinz Ploughman's	133	0.9	31.8	0.2	1.1
Tangy Tomato Cup Noodle	Golden Wonder	416	8.7	62.2	14.7	n/a
Taramasalata		446	3.2	4.1	46.4	N

Tartare Sauce	Burgess	285	1.9	19.3	21.5	0.7
	Colman's	272	1.3	16.0	20.0	n/a
Teacakes	Tunnock's	413	5.2	61.0	18.1	n/a
Teacakes, toasted		329	8.9	58.3	8.3	N
Teatime Mallows	Jacob's	389	3.9	64.9	12.7	2.4
Tendercrisp Corn	Green Giant	65.0	2.6	14.4	0.5	1.8
Tequila Sunrise, per pack	Boots Shapers	47.0	n/a	n/a	nil	n/a
Teriyaki Stir Fry Sauce	Sharwood	91.0	0.9	19.7	1.0	0.3
Texan Hot Chilli Pots of the World	Golden Wonder	399	11.1	57.6	13.8	n/a
Texas Hot American Sauce	Heinz	69.0	1.2	15.4	0.2	0.6
Thai Chicken & Lemon Grass Soup of the World	Knorr	333	9.0	63.6	4.7	n/a
Thai Cook-In-Sauce	Homepride	130	1.8	10.1	9.2	n/a
Thai Curry Sauce & Vegetables Stir Fry	Uncle Ben's	91.0	1.3	11.7	4.4	n/a

All amounts given per 100g/100ml unless otherwise stated

Product	*Brand*	*Calories kcal*	*Protein (g)*	*Carbo-hydrate (g)*	*Fat (g)*	*Dietary Fibre (g)*
Thai Hot Curry Paste	Sharwood	222	5.4	11.2	17.3	5.5
Thai Prawn Molee	Heinz Weight Watchers	89.0	3.8	13.7	2.1	0.7
Thai Special Fried Savoury Rice, per packet, as served	Batchelors	481	10.5	94.1	6.9	6.2
Thick Country Vegetable with Ham Soup	Heinz	64.0	3.0	8.2	2.0	1.0
Thomas the Tank Engine Spaghetti	Heinz	59.0	1.9	11.9	0.4	0.6
Thousand Island Dressing	Kraft	393	1.0	14.0	37.0	1.0
fat free	Kraft	98.0	0.6	25.5	Tr	2.5
low fat	Heinz Weight Watchers	79.0	1.7	8.3	4.3	0.1
Thousand Island Prawnnaise	Lyons Seafoods	405	6.3	3.0	41.6	n/a
Thread Noodles	Sharwood	322	11.5	69.2	1.9	3.4
Three Fruits Marmalade	Baxters	200	Tr	53.0	Tr	0.1

Tiffin	Cadbury	485	7.5	60.0	23.8	n/a
Tiger King Prawns, cooked	Lyons Seafoods	61.0	13.5	nil	0.6	n/a
Tiger Prawns, headless + shell	Lyons Seafoods	84.0	19.6	nil	0.7	n/a
Tikka Curry Paste	Sharwood	163	3.9	7.6	13.0	4.2
Tikka Masala Casserole Mix, as sold	Colman's	385	7.7	56.0	14.0	n/a
Tikka Masala Classic Curry Sauce	Homepride	85.0	2.0	7.4	5.2	n/a
Tikka Masala Cook-In-Sauce	Homepride	90.0	2.2	13.7	3.9	n/a
Tikka Masala Curry Sauce	Sharwood	99.0	3.0	8.4	5.8	2.3
Tikka Prawnnaise Light	Lyons Seafoods	218	5.2	6.1	19.3	n/a
Time Out	Cadbury	540	7.1	55.0	32.3	n/a
Tip Top	Nestlé	112	4.8	9.0	6.3	n/a
Tiramisu	McVitie's	337	3.5	31.2	22.2	0.3
Tizer	Barr	41.0	n/a	n/a	Tr	Tr
diet	Barr	0.2	n/a	Tr	Tr	Tr

All amounts given per 100g/100ml unless otherwise stated

Product	Brand	Calories kcal	Protein (g)	Carbo-hydrate (g)	Fat (g)	Dietary Fibre (g)
Toast: ***see Bread***						
Toasted Crunchy Oatbran	Mornflake	383	16.2	62.6	9.3	18.5
Toasted Oat Crunchy	Mornflake	351	11.0	52.0	11.0	6.0
Toasted Sesame Pitta Bread	International Harvest	263	9.7	48.0	3.6	3.0
Toast Toppers (Heinz): ***see individual flavours***						
Toffee Bon Bons, each	Trebor Bassett	29.0	nil	5.6	0.6	nil
Toffee Cheesecake	Green's/ Homepride	342	3.2	37.5	19.3	n/a
Toffee Crisp	Nestlé	498	4.6	60.6	26.4	n/a
Toffee Crumble, each	Lyons Maid	170	1.9	19.6	9.3	n/a
Toffee Crusha	Burgess	195	nil	48.5	nil	nil
Toffee Cup Cakes	Lyons Bakeries	391	3.3	67.7	13.8	0.5
Toffee Mousse, each	Fiesta	78.0	1.8	9.6	3.8	n/a

Toffee Napoli	Lyons Maid	107	1.8	14.5	5.8	n/a
Toffees, mixed		430	2.1	71.1	17.2	nil
Toffee YoYo	McVitie's	476	5.3	66.9	20.9	1.0
Toffets	G. Payne & Co	484	4.5	67.0	22.0	n/a
Toffo	Nestlé	451	2.2	69.8	18.1	n/a
Tofu (soya bean curd)						
steamed		73.0	8.1	0.7	4.2	N
steamed, fried		261	23.5	2.0	17.7	N
Tomato & Basil Quick Serve Soup, as served	Batchelors	195	3.9	31.7	6.3	n/a
Tomato & Brown Lentil Soup	Baxters	39.0	2.4	8.7	0.1	1.5
Tomato & Herb Potatoes 'n' Sauce, as served	Batchelors	455	12.1	76.9	11.2	2.8
Tomato & Herb Stir & Serve Soup	Knorr	433	7.3	45.8	24.5	n/a
Tomato & Lentil Cup-A-Soup Special, per sachet	Batchelors	73.0	2.7	14.8	0.7	n/a

All amounts given per 100g/100ml unless otherwise stated

Product	*Brand*	*Calories kcal*	*Protein (g)*	*Carbo-hydrate (g)*	*Fat (g)*	*Dietary Fibre (g)*
Tomato & Lentil Slim-A-Soup Special, per sachet	Batchelors	54.0	2.9	10.0	0.5	n/a
Tomato & Lentil Soup	Heinz Wholesoup	54.0	2.8	10.2	0.2	0.9
Tomato & Onion Casserole Recipe Sauce	Knorr	71.0	1.3	10.9	2.8	n/a
Tomato & Onion Cook-In-Sauce	Homepride	55.0	1.1	10.6	0.7	n/a
Tomato & Onion Mello 'n' Mild	Colman's	128	3.1	n/a	2.1	n/a
Tomato & Orange Soup	Baxters	40.0	1.0	8.5	0.5	0.3
Tomato & Sausage Bronto's Monster Feet	McVitie's	208	8.4	28.9	7.3	n/a
Tomato & Smoky Bacon Pasta 'n' Sauce, as served	Batchelors	471	18.5	104.1	2.6	10.9
Tomato & Tarragon Low In						

Fat Sauce	Homepride	230	1.1	7.0	2.6	n/a
Tomato & Vegetable Cup-A-Soup Special, per sachet	Batchelors	100	2.1	17.1	3.0	n/a
Tomato & Vegetable Soup, per pack	Boots Shapers	37.00	n/a	n/a	0.6	n/a
Tomato, Bean & Vegetable Soup	Baxters	40.0	2.3	7.9	0.1	1.5
Tomato Chutney		161	1.2	40.9	0.4	1.4
	Baxters	148	1.6	37.2	0.2	0.9
Tomato Cup-A-Soup, per sachet	Batchelors	78.0	0.5	15.7	1.9	n/a
Tomatoes, raw		17.0	0.7	3.1	0.3	1.0
fried in oil		91.0	0.7	5.0	7.7	1.3
grilled		49.0	2.0	8.9	0.9	2.9
canned		16.0	1.0	3.0	0.1	0.7
cherry, raw		18.0	0.8	3.0	0.4	1.0
Tomato Fresco	Napolina	19.5	1.5	3.6	Tr	n/a

All amounts given per 100g/100ml unless otherwise stated

Product	Brand	Calories kcal	Protein (g)	Carbo-hydrate (g)	Fat (g)	Dietary Fibre (g)
Tomato, Garlic & Olive Pizza Topping	Napolina	73.0	1.7	9.3	3.0	n/a
Tomato Juice		14.0	0.8	3.0	Tr	0.6
	Napolina	16.0	0.7	3.4	Tr	n/a
Tomato Juice Cocktail	Britvic	25.0	0.3	11.7	Tr	n/a
Tomato Ketchup		98.0	2.1	24.0	Tr	0.9
	Crosse & Blackwell	125	1.0	28.2	0.1	0.2
	Daddies	118	1.2	27.0	0.6	n/a
	Heinz	101	1.3	23.8	0.1	0.8
	HP	119	1.3	26.1	1.0	n/a
Tomato Ketchup with Mild Curry Spices	Lea & Perrins	123	1.5	26.7	1.1	n/a
Tomato Low Calorie Soup	Knorr	360	9.0	53.0	12.4	n/a
Tomato Napoli Pasta Soup	Heinz	44.0	4.3	8.4	0.6	0.5
Tomato Noodle Soup	Knorr	336	10.0	62.4	5.1	n/a

Tomato, Onion & Herb Pasta 'n' Sauce	Batchelors	489	9.3	67.3	24.6	10.7
Tomato Pickle	Heinz Ploughman's	105	2.2	23.4	0.2	1.8
Tomato Puree		68.0	4.5	12.9	0.2	2.8
	Napolina	90.0	4.8	18.0	nil	n/a
Tomato Quick Soup	Knorr	379	5.5	65.6	10.5	n/a
Tomato Rice Soup	Campbell's	47.0	0.8	8.6	1.0	n/a
Tomato Sauce		89.0	2.2	8.6	5.5	1.4
	Burgess	156	1.8	34.7	Tr	1.3
Tomato Sauce Crisps, per pack	Golden Wonder	153	2.0	12.2	10.6	1.3
Tomato Soup, dried, as served		31.0	0.6	6.3	0.5	N
dried, as sold		321	6.6	65.0	5.6	N
low calorie	Heinz Weight Watchers	25.0	0.5	4.1	0.7	0.6
Tomato Supernaturals, per pack	Golden Wonder	93.0	1.0	10.6	5.1	0.2

All amounts given per 100g/100ml unless otherwise stated

Product	Brand	Calories kcal	Protein (g)	Carbo-hydrate (g)	Fat (g)	Dietary Fibre (g)
Tomato, Sweetcorn & Mushroom Pizza Topping	Napolina	87.0	2.0	13.5	2.6	n/a
Tomato with Mushrooms & Herbs Pasta Sauce	Buitoni	96.0	1.8	19.8	0.8	0.8
Tongue, canned		213	16.0	nil	16.5	nil
Tonic Water	Schweppes	21.8	n/a	5.1	n/a	n/a
Tooty Fruities	Nestlé	404	0.4	92.4	3.6	n/a
Top Deck	Cadbury	525	8.1	57.3	29.2	n/a
Topic	Mars	497	7.4	55.3	27.6	n/a
Toppas	Kellogg's	320	9.0	69.0	1.5	8.0
Tornado, each	Lyons Maid	61.0	nil	15.2	nil	n/a
Tortellini Italiana	Heinz Weight Watchers	62.0	2.0	9.4	1.8	0.6
Tortelloni 5 Cheese, as sold	Dolmio	334	14.7	44.6	10.7	n/a
Tortelloni Italian Ham, as sold	Dolmio	297	15.3	41.1	7.9	n/a

Tortelloni Mushroom & Garlic, as sold	Dolmio	275	10.3	45.2	5.8	n/a
Tortelloni Veg. Cheese, Garlic & Herbs, as sold	Dolmio	329	13.4	46.2	10.1	n/a
Tortilla Chips		459	7.6	60.1	22.6	4.9
Traditional Beef Casserole Mix, as sold	Colman's	309	9.9	60.0	2.5	n/a
Traditional Chicken Casserole Mix, as sold	Colman's	291	8.0	62.0	0.6	n/a
Traditional Crunchy Original Toasted Oats Cereal						
with bran & apple	Mornflake	380	11.0	52.0	12.0	14.0
with honey, almonds & raisins	Mornflake	390	12.0	60.0	11.5	14.0
with oat bran & nuts	Mornflake	361	10.5	60.0	12.0	12.0
Traditional Golden Pouring Syrup	Lyle's	284	Tr	76.0	nil	nil

All amounts given per 100g/100ml unless otherwise stated

Product	*Brand*	*Calories kcal*	*Protein (g)*	*Carbo-hydrate (g)*	*Fat (g)*	*Dietary Fibre (g)*
Traditional Herb Mustard	Colman's	212	8.2	22.0	9.0	n/a
Traditional Macaroni Cheese Pasta 'n' Sauce, as served	Batchelors	481	23.1	85.3	8.7	7.1
Traditional Malt Bakes	McVitie's	502	5.9	67.0	22.9	1.8
Traditional Ragu	Brooke Bond	79.0	1.9	12.1	2.8	n/a
Traditional Ragu Sauce	Batchelors	63.0	2.1	8.8	2.1	n/a
Traditional Rice Pudding with Sultanas & Nutmeg	Ambrosia	101	3.3	17.1	2.6	n/a
Traditional Sausage Casserole Cooking Mix	Colman's	321	13.0	62.0	1.6	n/a
Traditional Style Lemonade	Idris	26.0	Tr	7.0	Tr	n/a
Traditional Tomato & Herbs Pasta Sauce	Buitoni	105	1.8	21.7	0.9	0.5
Traditional Wholemeal Bread	Allinson	217	10.3	38.4	2.5	6.5
Traditional Xmas Pudding	Holland					

	& Barrett	307	3.9	59.7	7.5	nil
Trail Mix		432	9.1	37.2	28.5	4.3
Treacle, black		257	1.2	67.2	nil	nil
Treacle Lattice Tart	Mr Kipling	384	3.9	65.6	11.8	n/a
Treacle Sponge Pudding	Heinz	275	2.3	48.2	8.2	0.6
Treacle Tart		368	3.7	60.4	14.1	1.1
Treacle Tarts	Lyons Bakeries	414	4.0	66.5	14.5	1.3
Treasure Crunch	Mornflake	406	12.2	60.0	13.0	6.5
Trebor Mints, each	Trebor Bassett	6.3	nil	1.5	Tr	n/a
Trifle		160	3.6	22.3	6.3	0.5
Trifle Mix, all flavours, as sold	Bird's	415	2.8	77.0	10.5	0.8
Trifle Sponge	Lyons Bakeries	318	5.3	70.0	1.9	1.1
Trifle with Fresh Cream		166	2.4	19.5	9.2	0.5
Trio Biscuits	Jacob's	528	5.2	59.6	29.9	1.0

All amounts given per 100g/100ml unless otherwise stated

Product	*Brand*	*Calories kcal*	*Protein (g)*	*Carbo-hydrate (g)*	*Fat (g)*	*Dietary Fibre (g)*
Trio Choc Biscuits	Jacob's	521	5.6	58.8	29.3	1.9
Trio Mallows	Jacob's	455	3.7	71.3	17.2	0.4
Tripe, dressed		60.0	9.4	nil	2.5	nil
dressed, stewed		100	14.8	nil	4.5	nil
Triple Chocolate Fudge Premium Ice Cream	Heinz Weight Watchers	168	4.1	22.2	6.5	1.0
Triple Toffee Fudge Premium Ice Cream	Heinz Weight Watchers	161	3.1	23.9	5.4	nil
Triple X Mints	Nestlé	396	0.7	98.4	nil	n/a
Tropical Alpen	Weetabix	367	11.0	65.1	6.9	7.8
Tropical Coconut Club Class	Jacob's	527	5.9	5837	31.6	3.2
Tropical Fruit Burst	Del Monte	45.0	0.2	11.1	Tr	n/a
Tropical Fruit Dessert Bombes	Heinz Weight Watchers	117	0.9	21.1	2.1	5.3
Tropical Fruit Drink, per pack	Boots Shapers	nil	n/a	n/a	nil	n/a

Tropical Fruit Solar	McVitie's	456	6.1	56.5	22.9	1.8
Tropical Juice Bar, each	Lyons Maid	37.0	Tr	9.9	Tr	n/a
Tropical Mix	Ross	64.0	2.5	9.5	2.8	2.4
Tropical Prawns	Lyons Seafoods	51.0	12.0	nil	0.5	n/a
cooked & peeled	Lyons Seafoods	53.0	12.0	nil	0.6	n/a
in brine	Lyons Seafoods	71.0	14.3	2.0	0.7	n/a
Tropical Special R Ready to Drink Carton	Robinsons	5.0	0.1	0.8	Tr	n/a
Tropical Squash, undiluted	St Clements	186	0.3	44.4	0.2	n/a
Trout, brown, steamed, flesh only		135	23.5	nil	4.5	nil
Tuc Biscuits	McVitie's	530	7.1	60.8	28.1	2.1
Tuc Savoury Sandwich Biscuits	McVitie's	571	8.0	49.5	37.5	1.5
Tuna						
canned in oil, drained		189	27.1	nil	9.0	nil
canned in brine, drained		99.0	23.5	nil	0.6	nil

All amounts given per 100g/100ml unless otherwise stated

Product	*Brand*	*Calories kcal*	*Protein (g)*	*Carbo-hydrate (g)*	*Fat (g)*	*Dietary Fibre (g)*
Tuna & Mayonnaise Pâté	Shippams	239	18.5	0.7	18.0	n/a
Tuna & Pasta Bake Casserole Mix, as sold	Colman's	3.4	11.0	54.0	4.9	n/a
Tuna & Tomato Club Sandwiches, per pack	Boots Shapers	189	n/a	n/a	n/a	n/a
Tuna & Tomato Spread, per pack	Boots Shapers	90.0	n/a	n/a	2.9	n/a
Tuna Chunks/Steaks						
Canned in Brine	Heinz	99.0	23.5	nil	0.6	nil
Canned in Vegetable Oil	Heinz	189	27.1	nil	9.0	nil
Tuna Crumble	Ross	191	7.5	14.4	11.9	0.6
Tuna in Mayonnaise Sandwich Maker	Shippams	178	14.0	2.2	12.6	n/a
Tuna Mayonnaise with Cucumber Sandwiches, per pack	Boots Shapers	199	n/a	n/a	n/a	n/a

Tuna Sandwich Filler	Heinz	189	6.2	10.2	13.7	0.2
Tuna Twists Shells Italiana	Heinz Weight Watchers	60.0	4.1	7.9	1.4	0.5
Tunes	Mars	392	nil	98.1	nil	n/a
Turkey, roast						
meat only		140	28.8	nil	2.7	nil
meat & skin		171	28.0	nil	6.5	nil
light meat		132	29.8	nil	1.4	nil
dark meat		148	27.8	nil	4.1	nil
Turkey & Bacon Bap, each	Boots Shapers	195	n/a	n/a	n/a	n/a
Turkey & Chinese Leaf with Sage & Onion Mayonnaise Sandwiches, per pack	Boots Shapers	183	n/a	n/a	n/a	n/a
Turkey & Ham Bap, each	Boots Shapers	191	n/a	n/a	n/a	n/a
Turkey, Ham & Coleslaw Sandwiches, per pack	Boots Shapers	231	n/a	n/a	n/a	n/a
Turkish Delight	Cadbury	525	2.1	69.0	30.1	n/a
per pack	Boots Shapers	98.0	n/a	n/a	3.5	n/a

All amounts given per 100g/100ml unless otherwise stated

Product	*Brand*	*Calories kcal*	*Protein (g)*	*Carbo-hydrate (g)*	*Fat (g)*	*Dietary Fibre (g)*
Turkish Delight without nuts		295	0.6	77.9	nil	nil
Turnip, boiled		12.0	0.6	2.0	0.2	1.9
Twiglets	Jacob's	394	12.1	61.4	11.0	6.8
Twinpack Oatcake, per pack	Boots Shapers	n/a	n/a	n/a	3.6	n/a
Twirl	Cadbury	525	8.1	55.9	30.1	n/a
Twix	Mars	495	5.8	63.5	24.2	n/a
Tzatziki		66.0	3.7	2.0	4.9	0.2

U

Ultra Light Very Low Fat Dairy Spread with Cheese	Primula	36.0	n/a	n/a	n/a	n/a
Um Bongo Fruit Drink	Libby	43.0	Tr	10.7	Tr	Tr
Uncle Ben's Stir Fry Range: *see individual flavours*						
United Biscuits						
golden crunch	McVitie's	499	5.9	64.7	23.4	1.5
mint	McVitie's	499	5.8	67.0	23.1	1.5
orange	McVitie's	498	5.8	64.6	23.3	1.5
Unsalted Rice Cakes	Holland & Barrett	376	8.5	77.2	3.1	7.5
Unsweetened Soya Milk	Holland & Barrett	37.0	3.6	0.6	2.1	Tr

All amounts given per 100g/100ml unless otherwise stated

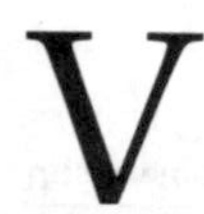

Product	Brand	Calories kcal	Protein (g)	Carbo-hydrate (g)	Fat (g)	Dietary Fibre (g)
Vanilla & Toffee Sundae, per pack	Boots Shapers	118	n/a	n/a	4.2	n/a
Vanilla Blancmange Powder, as sold	Brown & Polson	341	0.6	83.0	0.7	n/a
Vanilla Creme de Creme, each	Lyons Maid	166	3.0	21.3	8.3	n/a
Vanilla Creme Yogurt	St Ivel Shape	40.0	4.5	5.2	0.1	nil
Vanilla Cup, each	Lyons Maid	181	3.3	25.5	8.1	n/a
Vanilla Dairy Ice Cream	Heinz Weight Watchers	142	3.1	18.8	5.5	nil
Vanilla Flavour Dessert with						

Caramel Sauce	Chambourcy	108	3.3	22.8	0.8	Tr
Vanilla Flavour Rice	Ambrosia	101	3.3	16.0	2.7	n/a
Vanilla Fudge	Cravens	469	1.1	77.6	17.1	nil
Vanilla Fudge Hot Chocolate, per pack	Boots Shapers	40.0	n/a	n/a	0.9	n/a
Vanilla Ice Cream	Fiesta	155	3.6	19.2	7.6	n/a
	Lyons Maid	87.0	1.7	11.0	4.5	n/a
per pack	Boots Shapers	83.0	n/a	n/a	3.3	n/a
Vanilla King Cone, each	Lyons Maid	174	2.8	23.6	7.6	n/a
Vanilla Mr Men, each	Lyons Maid	52.0	1.2	8.8	1.4	n/a
Vanilla Napoli	Lyons Maid	100	1.9	10.6	5.6	n/a
Vanilla Soft Serve Ice Cream	Fiesta	161	3.3	19.4	8.3	n/a
Vanilla Walnut Whip	Nestlé	492	5.8	60.6	25.1	n/a
Vanilla Yogurt	St Ivel Shape	40.0	4.5	5.3	0.1	nil
Veal						
cutlet, fried in oil		215	31.4	4.4	8.1	0.1
fillet, roast		230	31.6	nil	11.5	nil

All amounts given per 100g/100ml unless otherwise stated

Product	*Brand*	*Calories kcal*	*Protein (g)*	*Carbo-hydrate (g)*	*Fat (g)*	*Dietary Fibre (g)*
Vegetable & Beef Slim-A-Soup, per sachet	Batchelors	37.0	1.2	7.9	0.3	n/a
Vegetable Au Gratin	Heinz Weight Watchers	94.0	3.9	12.1	3.3	1.0
Vegetable Bake	Ross	80.0	2.4	13.0	2.9	1.9
Vegetable Bolognese	Holland & Barrett	345	22.4	49.2	6.5	9.5
Vegetable Burger Mix	Holland & Barrett	158	8.3	13.6	7.8	4.3
Vegetable Burgers, each	Birds Eye Steakhouse	85.0	7.0	·5.0	4.0	2.3
Vegetable Casserole	Holland & Barrett	39.0	2.0	6.9	0.3	0.7
Vegetable Chilli	Holland & Barrett	65.0	4.8	11.6	0.3	2.8
	Homepride	52.0	1.2	10.9	0.4	n/a

per pack	Birds Eye Menu Master	315	8.5	64.0	2.5	4.2
Vegetable Chilli with Rice	Heinz Weight Watchers	84.0	2.9	14.2	1.7	0.8
per pack	Birds Eye Menu Master	460	9.0	68.0	17.0	4.2
Vegetable Curry	Holland & Barrett	375	22.3	45.1	10.8	8.9
	Tyne Brand	57.0	2.0	9.6	1.4	n/a
Vegetable Feasts, each	Birds Eye Country Club	105	2.0	13.0	5.0	1.7
Vegetable Ghee	Sharwood	897	Tr	Tr	99.7	nil
Vegetable Goulash	Holland & Barrett	41.0	1.3	7.8	0.5	0.8
Vegetable Granules, as sold	Oxo	297	8.8	57.4	5.2	n/a
Vegetable Gravy Granules, as sold	Brooke Bond	297	8.8	57.4	5.2	n/a

All amounts given per 100g/100ml unless otherwise stated

Product	*Brand*	*Calories kcal*	*Protein (g)*	*Carbo-hydrate (g)*	*Fat (g)*	*Dietary Fibre (g)*
Vegetable Hotpot	Heinz Weight Watchers	76.0	3.4	10.0	2.5	1.0
Vegetable Hot Pot Simply Fix Dry Mix, as sold	Crosse & Blackwell	325	15.3	49.6	7.3	1.3
Vegetable Korma Soup	Baxters	43.0	1.5	8.3	0.7	1.4
Vegetable Lasagne	Heinz Weight Watchers	74.0	4.6	10.5	1.7	0.9
	Ross	110	5.3	12.6	4.7	0.9
Vegetable Lasagne Microchef Meal	Batchelors	92.0	4.4	13.8	2.7	n/a
Vegetable Moussaka	Heinz Weight Watchers	68.0	2.5	9.1	2.4	0.3
Vegetable Oil		899	Tr	nil	99.9	nil
Vegetable Oxo Cubes	Brooke Bond	266	11.5	40.9	6.3	n/a
Vegetable Pasta Medley	Birds Eye Menu Master	170	6.5	23.0	5.5	4.1

Vegetable Pie	Ross	246	5.1	27.5	13.9	2.5
Vegetable Ravioli	Crosse & Blackwell	63.0	1.8	13.0	0.4	0.4
Vegetable Ravioli with Tomato Sauce Italiana	Heinz Weight Watchers	68.0	1.6	10.9	2.1	0.5
Vegetable Rice & Things Dry Mix, as sold	Crosse & Blackwell	360	8.5	76.1	2.4	3.7
Vegetable Risotto	Findus Lean Cuisine	94.0	2.9	14.9	2.5	1.5
Vegetable Salad	Heinz	150	1.4	14.7	9.5	1.6
Vegetable Samosas: *see Samosas*						
Vegetable Sausage Mix	Holland & Barrett	151	7.2	11.2	8.6	4.3
Vegetables Caribbean	Del Monte	71.0	3.5	8.8	2.5	n/a
Vegetables Cantonese	Del Monte	74.0	1.3	11.7	2.5	n/a
Vegetables Mexican	Del Monte	116	5.6	14.3	4.0	n/a

Product	Brand	Calories kcal	Protein (g)	Carbo-hydrate (g)	Fat (g)	Dietary Fibre (g)
Vegetable Soup, canned, ready to serve		37.0	1.5	6.7	0.7	1.5
	Campbell's	30.0	0.8	6.3	0.2	n/a
	Heinz	42.0	1.2	7.6	0.8	0.9
	Heinz Weight Watchers	25.0	0.9	4.5	0.3	0.7
Vegetables South Sea Island	Del Monte	86.0	1.9	12.0	3.4	n/a
Vegetable Stock Cubes	Knorr	327	12.3	27.0	18.9	n/a
Vegetable Sweet & Sour	Holland & Barrett	36.0	1.5	6.8	0.2	0.9
Vegetable Tikka Masala with Rice	Heinz Weight Watchers	84.0	2.5	14.0	2.0	0.4
Vegetarian Double Gloucester Cheese	Holland & Barrett	405	24.6	0.1	34.0	n/a
Vegetarian Mild Cheddar Cheese	Holland & Barrett	412	25.5	0.1	34.4	n/a

Vegetarian Mincemeat	Holland & Barrett	255	0.5	61.8	2.3	2.3
Vegetarian Red Leicester Cheese	Holland & Barrett	401	24.3	0.1	33.7	n/a
Venison, roast, meat only		198	35.0	nil	6.4	nil
Vermouth						
dry		118	0.1	5.5	nil	nil
sweet		151	Tr	15.9	nil	nil
Very Low Fat Spread		273	8.3	3.6	25.0	nil
Vessen Pâté: *see individual flavours*						
Vice Versas	Nestlé	487	6.1	67.5	21.4	n/a
Vichyssoise	Crosse & Blackwell	54.0	1.2	5.9	2.8	0.3
Victoria Sponge Mix	Green's	367	6.0	52.0	15.0	n/a
Viennese Biscuit	Holland & Barrett	537	4.1	60.9	30.8	nil
Viennese Whirls	Lyons Bakeries	512	4.1	55.1	30.6	1.3

All amounts given per 100g/100ml unless otherwise stated

Product	*Brand*	*Calories kcal*	*Protein (g)*	*Carbo-hydrate (g)*	*Fat (g)*	*Dietary Fibre (g)*
Vinaigrette Dressing						
low fat	Heinz Weight Watchers	31.0	0.4	7.3	nil	0.1
fat free	Kraft	40.0	Tr	10.0	Tr	0.7
Vindaloo Classic Curry Sauce	Homepride	56.0	1.9	8.8	0.3	n/a
Vintage Cider: ***see Cider***						
Vintage Orange Marmalade	Baxters	210	Tr	53.0	Tr	0.8
Vitbe Bread, etc.: ***see individual flavours***						
Vodka: ***see Spirits***						

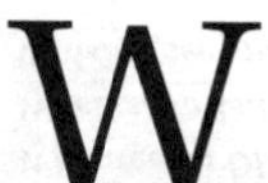

Wafer Biscuits, filled		535	4.7	66.0	29.9	N
Wafer Cream	Tunnock's	513	6.6	63.2	28.0	n/a
Waffles: ***see Potato Waffles***						
Waistline Oil-Free French Dressing	Crosse & Blackwell	11.0	0.7	0.3	0.2	0.1
Waistline Oil-Free Vinaigrette	Crosse & Blackwell	13.0	0.7	0.7	0.2	0.2
Waistline Reduced Calorie Dressing	Crosse & Blackwell	140	0.8	11.0	9.9	0.3
Walnut Halves	Holland & Barrett	662	13.4	3.3	65.0	6.6
	Whitworths	525	10.6	5.0	51.5	5.2

Product	*Brand*	*Calories kcal*	*Protein (g)*	*Carbo-hydrate (g)*	*Fat (g)*	*Dietary Fibre (g)*
Walnuts		688	14.7	3.3	68.5	3.5
Water Chestnuts, canned		31.0	0.9	7.4	Tr	N
Watermelon: ***see Melon***						
Weetabix	Weetabix	342	11.8	67.8	2.7	10.1
Weetaflakes	Weetabix	351	10.0	72.1	2.5	9.2
Weetos	Weetabix	385	6.3	78.8	4.9	5.5
Weight Watchers Products (Heinz): ***see individual flavours***						
Wensleydale Cheese		377	23.3	0.1	31.5	nil
Wheat Flour: ***see Flour, wheat***						
Wheatgerm		302	26.7	44.7	9.2	15.6
Wheatgerm Bread	Vitbe	232	10.4	39.6	3.6	4.2
Wheatgerm Oil		899	Tr	nil	99.9	nil
Whelks, boiled, weighed with shells		14.0	2.8	Tr	0.3	nil
Whisky: ***see Spirits***						

Whitebait, fried		525	19.5	5.3	47.5	0.2
	Young's	96.0	15.4	nil	3.8	nil
White Bread: ***see also Bread***	Heinz Weight Watchers	231	10.6	43.6	1.6	2.8
	Hovis	237	9.5	44.4	2.4	2.5
	Mothers Pride	229	8.0	45.6	1.6	3.0
	Nimble	235	8.2	45.7	2.2	4.3
	Sunblest	230	7.6	46.3	1.6	2.3
White Cap Cooking Fat	Van Den Berghs	900	nil	nil	100	n/a
White Chocolate		529	8.0	58.3	30.9	nil
White Chocolate Buttons	Cadbury	535	8.8	56.5	30.3	n/a
White Chocolate Chip Harvest Chewy Bar, each	Quaker	103	1.6	15.9	3.3	0.6
White Chocolate Dessert Pot	Ambrosia	115	3.4	19.3	2.9	n/a
White Chocolate Mini Logs	Mr Kipling	139	1.5	18.4	6.5	n/a
White Chocolate Mini Rolls	Mr Kipling	136	1.4	17.9	6.4	n/a
White Flora	Van Den Berghs	900	nil	nil	100	nil

Product	*Brand*	*Calories kcal*	*Protein (g)*	*Carbo-hydrate (g)*	*Fat (g)*	*Dietary Fibre (g)*
White Pepper: *see Peppers*						
White Pitta Bread	International Harvest	251	8.6	50.0	1.8	2.3
White Pudding		450	7.0	36.3	31.8	N
White Rice: *see Rice*						
White Rolls: *see Bread Rolls*						
White Sauce						
savoury, made with whole milk		150	4.1	10.9	7.8	0.2
savoury, made with semi-skimmed milk		128	4.2	11.1	10.3	0.2
sweet, made with whole milk		170	3.8	18.6	9.5	0.2
sweet, made with semi-skimmed milk		150	3.9	18.8	7.2	0.2
White Sauce Mix, as sold	Colman's	371	11.0	58.0	9.9	n/a
White Stick, each	Nestlé	271	3.7	24.2	17.8	n/a
White Stilton Cheese: *see Stilton*						
White Wine						

dry		66.0	0.1	0.6	nil	nil
medium		75.0	0.1	3.4	nil	nil
sparkling		76.0	0.2	5.9	nil	nil
sweet		94.0	0.2	5.9	nil	nil
White Wine & Garlic Vinaigrette	Lea & Perrins	107	0.8	23.1	1.1	n/a
White Wine Casserole Recipe Sauce	Knorr	81.0	1.8	7.8	4.9	n/a
White Wine Cook-In-Sauce	Homepride	72.0	1.1	7.6	4.1	n/a
White Wine Pour Over Sauce	Baxters	130	3.0	8.1	9.4	0.1
Whiting						
steamed, flesh only		92.0	20.9	nil	0.9	nil
in crumbs, fried		191	18.1	7.0	10.3	0.3
Whole Dried Figs	Holland & Barrett	213	3.6	52.9	Tr	18.5
Wholegrain Mustard	Colman's	173	8.5	8.5	11.1	n/a

All amounts given per 100g/100ml unless otherwise stated

Product	*Brand*	*Calories kcal*	*Protein (g)*	*Carbo-hydrate (g)*	*Fat (g)*	*Dietary Fibre (g)*
Wholegrain Rice						
as sold	Uncle Ben's	340	8.9	70.8	2.4	n/a
frozen	Uncle Ben's	147	3.7	30.9	1.8	n/a
3 minute	Uncle Ben's	164	3.9	33.4	1.6	n/a
Wholemeal Bread	Nimble	226	13.8	36.1	3.0	5.8
Wholemeal Crackers		413	10.1	72.1	11.3	4.4
Wholemeal Crispbread	Allinson	355	13.2	68.2	3.3	9.8
Wholemeal Flour: *see Flour, wholemeal*						
Wholemeal Lambourn Scooples, each	Kavli	22.0	n/a	n/a	n/a	n/a
Wholemeal Loaf	Holland & Barrett	225	10.0	42.8	2.7	9.0
Wholemeal Malt Loaf	Allinson	259	10.6	48.2	2.6	6.8
Wholemeal Muffins, each	Allinson	145	7.8	25.5	1.4	4.0
Wholemeal Pastry: *see Pastry*						

Wholemeal Pitta Bread	International Harvest	226	11.7	39.8	2.2	6.4
Wholemeal Rolls	Holland & Barrett	232	10.0	43.0	2.7	9.0
each	Allinson	104	5.0	16.5	2.0	2.5
Wholemeal Scones: ***see Scones***						
Whole Milk: ***see Milk***						
Wholenut Chocolate	Cadbury	520	7.8	56.8	29.3	n/a
Wholenut Peanut Butter	Sunpat	620	13.1	4.8	10.2	0.4
Wholenut Tasters	Cadbury	555	9.9	44.2	37.8	n/a
Wholewheat Macaroni: ***see Macaroni***						
Wholewheat Ravioli: ***see Ravioli***						
Wholewheat Spaghetti: ***see Spaghetti***						
Wild Blackberry Jelly	Baxters	210	Tr	53.0	Tr	1.4
Wildlife	Cadbury	520	7.8	56.8	29.3	n/a
Wild Rowan Jelly	Baxters	252	Tr	67.0	Tr	1.5

	Brand	Calories kcal	Protein (g)	Carbo-hydrate (g)	Fat (g)	Dietary Fibre (g)
w/Willow Lightly Salted	Dairy Crest	709	0.7	1.0	78.0	n/a
ne: *see Red, Rosé, White*						
Wine Gums, each	Trebor Bassett	16.0	0.3	3.6	nil	nil
Winkles, boiled, weighed with shells		14.0	2.9	Tr	0.3	nil
Winter Vegetable Soup	Heinz Wholesoup	43.0	2.4	7.8	0.2	0.9
Winter Vegetable Wholesome Soup	Heinz Weight Watchers	32.0	1.4	6.1	0.2	1.1
Wispa	Cadbury	540	7.0	53.8	33.2	n/a
Wonderloaf	Mothers Pride	240	7.1	51.6	1.9	2.7
Woodpecker Cider	H P Bulmer	30.4	n/a	n/a	n/a	n/a
Woppa Chews, each	Trebor Bassett	18.0	Tr	3.8	0.2	n/a
Worcester Ketchup	Lea & Perrins	115	1.5	25.7	0.6	n/a

Worcester Sauce Wheat Crunchies, per pack	Golden Wonder	179	3.6	20.3	9.3	1.0
Worcestershire Sauce	Lea & Perrins	93.0	1.2	20.9	0.5	n/a

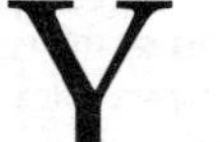

Yam, raw		114	1.5	28.2	0.3	1.3
boiled		133	1.7	33.0	0.3	1.4
Yeast, bakers, compressed		53.0	11.4	1.1	0.4	N
dried		169	35.6	3.5	1.5	N
Yellow Bean Stir Fry Sauce	Sharwood	129	0.3	28.9	1.7	1.5
Yellow Split Peas	Whitworths	310	22.1	56.6	1.0	5.9

Product	Brand	Calories kcal	Protein (g)	Carbo-hydrate (g)	Fat (g)	Dietary Fibre (g)
Yogurt						
Greek style, cows		115	6.4	2.0	9.1	nil
Greek style, sheep		106	4.4	5.6	7.5	nil
low calorie		41.0	4.3	6.0	0.2	N
low fat, plain		56.0	5.1	7.5	0.8	N
low fat, flavoured		90.0	3.8	17.9	0.9	N
low fat, fruit		90.0	4.1	17.9	0.7	N
soya		72.0	5.0	3.9	4.2	N
whole milk, plain		79.0	5.7	7.8	3.0	N
whole milk, fruit		105	5.1	15.7	2.8	N
Yogurt & Herb Dressing	Kraft	320	1.5	7.8	31.5	0.2
Yogurt & Herb Low Fat Dressing	Heinz Weight Watchers	76.0	2.5	7.2	4.2	nil
Yorkie (Rowntree Mackintosh): ***see individual flavours***						
Yorkshire Pudding		208	6.6	24.7	9.9	0.9

Young Broad Beans, 1oz/28g	Birds Eye	17.0	2.0	2.0	0.1	1.1
Young Sweetcorn, 1oz/28g	Birds Eye	33.0	1.0	6.0	0.5	0.5
YoYo (McVitie's): ***see individual flavours***						

Z

Zoom, each	Lyons Maid	46.0	0.3	10.0	0.5	n/a
Zucchini: ***see Courgettes***						
Zucchini Lasagne	Findus Lean Cuisine	64.0	5.0	7.9	1.4	1.6

COLLINS GEM

Bestselling Collins Gem titles include:

Gem English Dictionary (£3.50)
Gem Calorie Counter (£2.99)
Gem Thesaurus (£2.99)
Gem French Dictionary (£3.50)
Gem German Dictionary (£3.50)
Gem Burns Anthology (£3.50)
Gem Birds (£3.50)
Gem Babies' Names (£3.50)
Gem Card Games (£3.50)
Gem World Atlas (£3.50)

All Collins Gems are available from your local bookseller or can be ordered direct from the publishers.

In the UK, contact Mail Order, Dept 2M, HarperCollins Publishers, Westerhill Rd, Bishopbriggs, Glasgow, G64 2QT, listing the titles required and enclosing a cheque or p.o. for the value of the books plus £1.00 for the first title and 25p for each additional title to cover p&p. Access and Visa cardholders can order on 041-772 2281 (24 hr).

In Australia, contact Customer Services, HarperCollins Distribution, Yarrawa Rd, Moss Vale 2577 (tel. [048] 68 0300). **In New Zealand**, contact Customer Services, HarperCollins Publishers, 31 View Rd, Glenfield, Auckland 10 (tel. [09] 444 3740). **In Canada**, contact your local bookshop.

All prices quoted are correct at time of going to press.